The
Low-Starch
Diabetes Solution

Six Steps to Optimal Control of Your Adult-Onset (Type 2)
Diabetes with the Science of Insulin Resistance
and the Glycemic Load

ROB THOMPSON, M.D.

RECIPES BY
DANA CARPENDER

Mc
Graw
Hill

New York   Chicago   San Francisco   Lisbon   London   Madrid   Mexico City
Milan   New Delhi   San Juan   Seoul   Singapore   Sydney   Toronto

The *McGraw·Hill* Companies

Library of Congress Cataloging-in-Publication Data

Thompson, Rob, 1945–
    The low-starch diabetes solution : six steps to reduce insulin resistance and
your adult-onset (type 2) diabetes with the science of the glycemic load / by Rob
Thompson ; with low-starch recipes by Dana Carpender.
        p.   cm.
    Includes bibliographical references and index.
    ISBN 0-07-162150-2 (alk. paper)
        1. Non-insulin-dependent diabetes—Diet therapy—Recipes.   2. Low-
carbohydrate diet—Recipes.   3. Glycemic index.   4. Insulin
resistance.   I. Carpender, Dana.   II. Title.

    RC662.18. T46   2009
    616.4'620654—dc22   2009027017

Copyright © 2010 by Robert Thompson, M.D. All rights reserved. Printed in the United
States of America. Except as permitted under the United States Copyright Act of 1976,
no part of this publication may be reproduced or distributed in any form or by any
means, or stored in a database or retrieval system, without the prior written permission
of the publisher.

1 2 3 4 5 6 7 8 9 10 11 12 13 14 15 16 17 18 19 20 21 22   DOC/DOC   0 9

ISBN 978-0-07-162150-2
MHID   0-07-162150-4

McGraw-Hill books are available at special quantity discounts to use as premiums and
sales promotions or for use in corporate training programs. To contact a representative,
please e-mail us at bulksales@mcgraw-hill.com.

Contents

Part 2   Six Steps to Optimal Control of Your Diabetes

Part 3   Low-Starch Cuisine: Discovering a Tastier Way to Eat

Introduction

Until recently, doctors thought adult-onset diabetes was the same as childhood diabetes—that both were caused by lack of insulin. In the 1980s, scientists made the remarkable discovery that they're entirely different diseases. Whereas kids with diabetes lack insulin, most adult-onset diabetics make plenty of insulin—often more than normal. The problem is that their bodies lose sensitivity to it. Now doctors refer to the disease that young people get as type 1 diabetes and to the kind that middle-aged adults get as type 2-diabetes. *This book is for people with adult-onset, or type 2, diabetes.*

In times past, the diagnosis of diabetes had tragic implications. Children and young adults with type 1 diabetes often wasted away and died from it. Insulin, when it came along in the 1920s, was the miracle drug for these patients. It allowed them to live normal lives.

In those days, the troubles of middle-aged and older folks with type 2 diabetes seemed minor compared with young people with type 1 diabetes. Adult-onset diabetics could live for years with hardly any treatment at all. They could usually get their blood sugar down to reasonable levels by just taking some pills and watching their diet. Doctors rarely prescribed insulin for these patients; they figured it wasn't worth the trouble.

In the 1990s, new research showed that while patients with type 2 diabetes rarely died as a direct result of their diabetes, their

1

mildly elevated blood sugar levels—if these went on long enough—could result in damage to their eyes, kidneys, and blood vessels, and the attendant increase in heart attack rate was alarming. As a result, doctors started taking adult-onset diabetes more seriously, treating it as they would type 1 diabetes, using stronger pills and insulin when necessary to get blood sugar levels as close to normal as possible.

In 2008, researchers released the results of two large studies on the effects of this more vigorous approach to treating adult-onset diabetes. The results were disappointing. Heavier doses of insulin helped patients avoid eye and kidney damage but did little to reduce the rate of heart attacks. What worked for patients with juvenile diabetes didn't work as well for people with adult-onset diabetes.

Those results are not really surprising, considering that type 2 diabetes is a completely different disease from type 1. It has different causes, results in different complications, and requires a different approach to treatment. The goal of treating type 1 diabetes is simple: replace the missing insulin. Type 2 diabetes is more complicated. The body becomes resistant to the effects of insulin, which not only raises blood sugar but brings on cholesterol, blood pressure, and weight problems that cause as much trouble as the high blood sugar does. This often requires a multipronged approach to treatment.

The good news is that you can live to a ripe old age without suffering any health problems from your type 2 diabetes. When the nineteenth-century sage George Bernard Shaw said the secret to good health is to get a chronic disease and take good care of it, he might as well have been talking about adult-onset diabetes. When you do what you need to do to treat it, you reverse many of our modern lifestyle's harmful effects on your health and general well-being. Indeed, you might find yourself feeling better than you have for years.

This book will give you six simple steps to follow that should give you excellent control of your type 2 diabetes. First, however, it is important to understand the logic behind its treatment. Once you see what brought on your condition, you will know exactly what you need to do to reverse it.

Part 1

The Toxin

1

A Gift from
the Fertile Crescent

About ten thousand years ago, something happened near the eastern edge of the Mediterranean Sea that changed the course of history. Like all prehistoric people, the inhabitants of that region were hunter-gatherers. They lived on wild game and vegetation. However, they had become so efficient at hunting animals and gathering vegetation that they began to deplete their food supply. To thrive, they needed a new source of calories. They found one in an area that encompassed parts of modern Syria and Iraq known as the Fertile Crescent.

The Fertile Crescent had a unique climate. The summers were so hot and dry that they were deadly for most vegetation, but the winters were temperate and moist—ideal for plant growth. Those conditions fostered the evolution of a particular kind of plant, one that could mature fast enough during short growing seasons to drop its seeds before being killed by the scorching summers. The wild ancestors of wheat and barley flourished in the Fertile Crescent. The secret of their success was their seeds.

Wheat and barley seeds were loaded with *starch,* a white powder that provides energy for seeds to grow into sprouts. The unusually large amounts of starch in these seeds helped jump-start seedlings so they could mature quickly enough during the short growing seasons to drop the next generation of seeds before the dry season set in. Tough husks protected the contents of the seeds from the scorching summer heat and from predators. Ideally suited to the climate of the Fertile Crescent, wild wheat and barley covered the plains of the region, producing copious amounts of starch-rich seeds.

Starch consists of hundreds of sugar molecules linked together to form long chains. Although Mother Nature actually intended starch to be used to provide energy for plant seedlings rather than animals, the intestinal enzymes of many animals, including humans, are capable of breaking the loose bonds that hold together the sugar molecules in starch and using that sugar as a source of calories. Indeed, the starch in wild wheat and barley seeds represented a potentially enormous source of calories for our prehistoric ancestors. The challenge was getting to it. The seeds were encased in impermeable husks designed to keep out predators.

Approximately ten thousand years ago, some resourceful humans in the Fertile Crescent figured out how to separate the contents of wheat and barley seeds from the husks by grinding the seeds between rocks and letting the wind blow away the chaff. Eventually they learned to make the kernels more palatable by pulverizing them into flour, mixing the flour with water to make dough, and cooking the dough into bread. This bit of crude technology gave them access to an endless source of calories that had never before been tapped.

The ability to use wheat and barley as a source of calories turned out to be far more than a way to supplement the hunter-gatherer diet. It spawned the beginning of Western civilization. Because the seeds of wheat and barley had evolved to withstand long periods of drought, they could be stored for months if kept dry. With access to a seemingly endless source of calories that could be stockpiled between growing seasons, humans in the Fertile Crescent no longer had to roam in search of food. Because they no longer had to disperse themselves to find food, they could take advantage of the benefits of living in communities. Having an abundant supply of calories allowed members of these early societies to engage in activities other than food production, such as governing and defending themselves and establishing armies of conquest. The agricultural way of life that began in the Fertile Crescent spawned a civilization that, along with its reliance on grain, ultimately took over the Middle East, Europe, and the New World.

Similar phenomena took place in two other parts of the world with similar climates and similar grains. Rice and millet became staples in the Far East, and corn became a staple in America before the arrival of Europeans. As in the Fertile Crescent, the cultivation of starches fostered agricultural civilizations that eventually dominated their respective regions of the world.

Thousands of years later, the natives in South America introduced European explorers to another rich source of starch, the potato. Although potatoes are roots rather than seeds, like other starches they can be grown in abundance and stored between growing seasons. Potatoes eventually became a staple of the European and American diets.

Of all the foods humans eat, starch provides by far the most calories for the least investment of land, labor, and capital. In most parts of the world, humans now depend on starch for their very survival. Wheat, rice, corn, and potatoes have come to provide most of the starch—indeed, most of the calories—for the majority of people in the world.

The shift from the hunter-gatherer diet of meat and wild vegetation to one consisting largely of starch represented a profound change in the chemical composition of the human diet. Modern humans consume *hundreds* of times more sugar molecules in the form of starch than their prehistoric ancestors did. Digestive and hormonal systems evolve over millions of years to handle foods specific to each species. Considering that humans didn't start eating significant amounts of starch until about ten thousand years ago—a brief period in the span of human existence—whatever genetic adaptations might be needed to accommodate that change have not had time to occur.

Is there a price to be paid for our newfound dependence on starch? That's something I didn't think about much until 1999.

2

Lowering Blood Sugar the Old-Fashioned Way

The diagnosis took me by surprise. My family and I were on a ski vacation in Idaho when I found myself waking up several times at night, thirsty and needing to urinate. There's nothing unusual about a fifty-four-year-old man getting up to use the bathroom or having a few sips of water before going back to bed, but I was waking up three or four times a night, and the thirst was compelling. I didn't want to just sip water—I wanted to guzzle it. I knew something was wrong, and I figured adult-onset diabetes was at the top of the list.

Until then, I hadn't considered myself a candidate for diabetes. It tends to run in families, and nobody in my family had it. Most adult-onset diabetics are overweight. I was carrying a few extra pounds, but I didn't think I was fat enough to be at risk. Nevertheless, I knew it was a possibility. As a preventive cardiologist, I treated lots of people with diabetes. I had analyzers in my office for checking blood sugar, so I promised myself to check my own as soon as I got home.

The first day back in the office, I skipped breakfast and had Nadine, my medical assistant, draw my blood. It's easy to diagnose diabetes. You measure your blood sugar. If it's high, you've got it; if it's not, you don't. Doctors define diabetes as a fasting blood sugar level higher than 125. I figured that if, indeed, I had early diabetes, my blood sugar might have crept over the line a little, maybe 160 or 170 at most.

I was about to enter an examination room to see a patient when Nadine stopped me and handed me the results. My blood sugar was 380.

I was dumbfounded. I had never had any serious medical problems, but there it was: not just a little elevated; it was sky high. How did I get in that condition without noticing anything? One minute I'm healthy; the next I'm a full-fledged diabetic. What a hassle! I had enough to worry about. The last thing I needed was a medical problem that would require a lifetime of discipline and vigilance. I wasn't sure I could rise to the challenge of watching my diet, checking my blood sugar, and taking medications for the rest of my life.

As a doctor, however, I had seen the complications of poorly controlled diabetes—kidney failure, amputated feet, vision loss. I knew what diabetes could do. If you don't take care of it, you suffer serious consequences. I realized I wasn't in any immediate danger, but I figured I was getting a glimpse of the likely mode of my demise. Gone for sure, I thought, were my chances of living to a ripe old age.

What Was Happening

Like all diabetics, I wasn't making enough insulin to keep my blood sugar down. Your intestines break down plant-based foods, *carbohydrates*, into the sugar glucose, which is absorbed into your bloodstream. To get out of your bloodstream and into cells that use it, glucose has to pass through the membranes that surround cells, but it can't do that without the hormone insulin.

Tiny clusters of cells in your *pancreas*, a large gland behind your stomach, make insulin. These cells, called *beta cells*, sense when the glucose levels in your blood rise, and secrete insulin into the bloodstream to lower it. Insulin opens tiny gates in cell membranes, which allow glucose to pass out of the blood and into cells.

Because I wasn't making enough insulin, glucose was building up in my blood.

Doctors classify diabetes as type 1 or type 2—a crucial distinction. Damage to the insulin-producing cells from an immune response to an infection causes type 1. Because this kind of diabetes usually starts in childhood, it's also called juvenile diabetes. In type 2, or adult-onset diabetes, the beta cells make plenty of insulin, but the body loses sensitivity to it. In the early stages, the beta cells actually make *more* insulin than normal to compensate for the body's loss of sensitivity to insulin. Eventually the beta cells literally wear out from overwork. When your insulin production can no longer keep up with demand, your blood sugar rises. Being middle-aged, I figured I had typical adult-onset, type 2 diabetes.

As for the thirst and increased urination I was having, when the glucose levels in your blood get too high, glucose overflows into your urine and pulls water along with it, which causes excessive urination, dehydration, and thirst. Although it's common knowledge that increased urination and thirst are symptoms of diabetes, your blood sugar has to rise above 230 or so—considerably above the normal of 125—before sugar spills into the urine. The dehydration symptoms I was having should have been a clue that my blood sugar was not just a little higher than normal but way over the line.

If your blood sugar gets too high—above 500 or so—and stays there for several days, it can cause life-threatening dehydration, acid buildup, and shock. That's unlikely to happen if you keep your levels below 300 or so, which most type 2 patients can do with minimal attention to their diet. Milder elevations often don't cause noticeable symptoms at all. People sometimes go for years without knowing they have diabetes.

In 1999, when I discovered my diabetes, doctors were able to keep patients' blood sugar levels low enough to avoid dehydration and shock. The challenge was to prevent damage to blood vessels. This is difficult because even mildly elevated blood sugar, if it goes on for a few years, can injure the delicate, small arteries of the body—the *microvasculature*—and damage the eyes, kidneys, and nerves. Preventing microvascular complications requires that blood sugar be kept at or near normal levels, which is more difficult than just keeping it low enough to prevent dehydration.

Diabetes can also damage the large arteries of the body and cause heart attacks and strokes, which are leading causes of death of Americans and Europeans. Actually, diabetes doesn't directly harm the large arteries so much as it accelerates damage from other causes such as high blood cholesterol, high blood pressure, and cigarette smoking. I didn't have any of those "risk factors," so at least for the time being, I didn't worry much about large-artery damage. My main concern was the microvascular complications—eye, kidney, and nerve damage.

My unabashedly high blood sugar was proof that my metabolism was seriously deranged. I knew I needed to act. In addition to taking medication, I was going to have to change my lifestyle. I figured my days of undisciplined eating were over. No longer could I enjoy whatever I wanted and let myself get out of shape. If I didn't get a handle on this problem, everything else in my life was jeopardized.

All of these things flashed through my mind as I stood in my office hallway, staring at my blood sugar number. That was ten years ago.

A Curse or a Blessing?

I can't honestly say I'm glad I have diabetes, but in some ways it has turned out to be a blessing. It has shown me the way to a healthier lifestyle. I'm happy to report that my diabetes has remained in excellent control. I have suffered no health consequences from it. I'm more active than ever, in decent physical shape, and twenty pounds lighter than I was before.

Diabetes is a disease of modern civilization, brought on and aggravated by the way we live. Indeed, the modern lifestyle does more than cause diabetes. It makes us fat, frail, stressed out, and prone to a number of other diseases. In doing what I needed to do to treat my diabetes, I discovered a more enjoyable way to live. Indeed, in many ways I'm healthier now than I would have been if I hadn't gotten diabetes.

Unfortunately, I can't say the same for most patients with type 2 diabetes. Surveys show that the majority of adult diabetics don't control their condition well enough to prevent long-term complications such as eye, kidney, and blood vessel disease. According to the American Diabetes Association, less than half of patients meet the association's standards for adequate control of their blood sugar levels. Less than a third of diabetics who should be taking medications for reducing cholesterol and blood pressure are actually taking them.

How well patients are able to control their blood sugar levels depends greatly on how well they've been educated about the disease. However, I have found that most patients don't understand what raises their blood sugar or what they need to do to lower it. It's tragic that so many diabetics suffer from eye, kidney, and blood vessel damage when these problems are completely preventable. No one should suffer from complications of diabetes.

As a preventive cardiologist, I had treated hundreds of patients with diabetes, but getting the disease myself changed my perspective toward it. Diabetics and their doctors exist in two different worlds. As a doctor, I was in a world that revolved around making diagnoses, ordering tests, and prescribing medications. I gave advice to diabetics about how lifestyle changes could help them, but I wasn't the one who had to live with those recommendations. That was *their world*. When I got diabetes, I entered that world. I had no difficulty deciding what medication to take or what laboratory test I needed, but every day, I found myself grappling with decisions about a more primal aspect of life: what to eat. Having the disease never let me forget that diabetes is a disturbance in the way the body handles food. When I started having to live with diabetes, I began to delve deeper into an aspect of the disease I hadn't paid enough attention to—the role of diet.

The Old-Fashioned Way of Controlling Blood Sugar

Before insulin medication was developed in the 1920s, young diabetics would dwindle away as a result of a kind of internal starvation. Their beta cells couldn't produce enough insulin, so their blood sugar levels would rise so high that much of the calories they consumed would flow right out in their urine. The only way diabetics could control their blood sugar was to shun carbohydrates, foods the digestive tract turns to glucose. However, when insulin became available, physicians stopped advising diabetics to avoid carbohydrates. When combined with insulin, carbohydrates helped them put on weight, which doctors regarded as a sign of improving health.

Until the 1970s, doctors made no distinction between type 1 and type 2 diabetes. Because they thought diabetes in adults was just a milder form of the kind children got, they figured—incorrectly—that these patients were also internally starved of glucose, even if they were overweight. Doctors thought that as long as their type 2 diabetic patients got enough insulin, they would actually benefit from eating carbohydrates. To make matters worse, when researchers discovered links between high blood levels of cholesterol and heart disease, doctors started telling patients to eat less fat and cholesterol, which encouraged them to eat even more carbohydrates.

When I started practicing medicine in the 1970s, I accepted the prevailing scientific wisdom that dietary cholesterol causes high blood cholesterol. Although my blood cholesterol levels were OK, I still tried to avoid cholesterol-containing foods. I ate plenty of carbohydrates, including starchy stuff like bread, pasta, potatoes, and rice. Most doctors at the time considered these "empty calories." They figured that while these foods didn't provide much in the way of vital nutrients, because they were free of fat and cholesterol, they didn't do you any harm.

By the time I got diabetes, I had been practicing cardiology long enough to know that Americans' fear of dietary cholesterol was overblown. New research showed that avoiding cholesterol-containing foods did not prevent heart attacks or even lower blood cholesterol levels much. As for myself, having seen the complications of poorly controlled diabetes, I was more concerned about my blood sugar than my cholesterol level. Consequently, I made a decision about my diet that turned out to be a good one. I took the old-fashioned approach to lowering blood sugar. I didn't worry about the cholesterol in food. Instead, I concentrated on eliminating carbohydrates. I put myself on a strict low-carbohydrate diet. I cut out flour products, potatoes, rice, sweets, milk, and sugar-containing fruits and vegetables—anything my digestive system turned to glucose.

The results were impressive and immediate. Within a few days, my blood sugar fell to safe levels and stayed there. I was no longer thirsty all of the time. I didn't have to get up several times a night to use the bathroom. My energy level improved noticeably.

As for my blood cholesterol readings, my bad cholesterol (LDL) level stayed the same, and my good cholesterol (HDL) level went up. The balance between my good and bad cholesterol—the most accurate predictor of blood vessel disease—looked better than ever. From the start, I chose to treat my diabetes the old-fashioned way, by avoiding all carbohydrates.

Then I learned about the *new* old-fashioned way.

3

Glycemic Load: The *New* Old-Fashioned Way

The day after I discovered my diabetes, I went to a drugstore and bought a *glucometer*, a handheld device for measuring blood sugar. These little gadgets have revolutionized diabetes treatment. In the old days, if you wanted your blood sugar checked, you had to go to a doctor's office, have your blood drawn, and wait a day or two for the doctor to call you back with the results. But a diabetic's blood sugar can go up or down a couple hundred points in a matter of hours. There was no practical way of keeping track of such fluctuations. You could test your urine at home, but sugar doesn't spill into your urine until your blood level reaches at least 230 or so. If you wanted to get your blood sugar levels lower than that, you were groping in the dark.

Now, for less than the price of a week's worth of diabetes pills, you can buy a glucometer and check your blood sugar yourself. You can tell exactly what your levels are doing, not just from day to day, but from hour to hour.

After a typical meal, your blood glucose rises abruptly, peaks in about thirty minutes, and then drifts back down over the course of three or four hours. Doctors refer to measurements taken after meals as *postprandial* readings. How high your blood sugar rises after eating varies widely depending on the kind of carbohydrate you eat, what you eat with it, the order in which you eat your food, and your activity level before and after the meal. Normally, your blood sugar measured two hours after eating should not be higher than 140.

Measurements taken after not eating for several hours, so-called *fasting* blood sugar levels, vary much less than ones taken after eating, which is why most doctors use fasting levels to gauge how well patients are controlling their diabetes. Ideally, your fasting blood sugar should be less than 125. Starting with a fasting level of 380, I apparently had a long way to go.

Most doctors are satisfied if their patients have normal *fasting* blood sugar levels. They don't worry much about readings taken soon after meals. These vary so much that many physicians tell their patients not to even bother checking them. Personally, however, I wanted my blood sugar levels normal at all times, not just when I hadn't eaten for several hours. Once I got my fasting blood sugar levels under control, I started doing something most diabetics at the time didn't do. I began checking my blood sugar after eating.

This was an eye-opening experience. Even though my fasting levels were normal or near normal most of the time, my after-meal readings were all over the map. Many reputedly healthful foods, even ones deemed acceptable by the American Diabetes Association, caused my blood sugar to skyrocket. A hamburger shot it up a couple hundred points. A few handfuls of corn chips did the same. The bran muffin I was having for breakfast drove it up a hundred points. Raisin bran cereal was even worse.

I thought, "No wonder doctors don't tell their patients to check their blood sugar levels after meals. You feel like you're living in a diabetic minefield!" However, the news wasn't all bad.

The Steak and the Two Slices of Bread

One night, shortly after I discovered my diabetes, I treated myself to a great meal—a twelve-ounce steak, Caesar salad, asparagus, baked potato with butter and sour cream, and some good chocolate for dessert. Having recently read that baked potatoes raise blood sugar, I pushed aside the white part of the potato and just ate the skin, slathered in butter and sour cream. I figured a heavy meal like that would drive up my blood sugar for sure, but when I checked my sugar afterward, I was surprised to find that it barely budged. I checked it twice. It was true; I had just eaten a huge, delicious meal, and my blood sugar hardly rose at all. What a morale booster! Maybe life with diabetes wasn't going to be so bad after all.

Later, I wondered why I had been so surprised. One of the first things you learn in medical school is that there are three kinds of foods: carbohydrates, fats, and protein. Carbohydrates come from plants. You get fats from animal products and fatty vegetables like nuts and olives. Most protein comes from eggs, meat, and dairy products. Each of the three kinds of food is composed of a different building block: carbohydrates are made of sugar, fats of fatty acids, and proteins of amino acids. Your digestive system breaks down each kind to its basic building blocks before it is absorbed into your bloodstream. Once these nutrients are in your blood, your body needs insulin to handle the glucose that carbohydrates release, but it doesn't need insulin to metabolize fat and protein, which is largely what my steak dinner contained.

I guess I knew all of that intellectually but not at a gut level. I figured Mae West was right when she said that everything she liked was illegal, immoral, or fattening. I thought having diabetes meant a lifetime of deprivation, but that's not so at all. The fact is this: *diabetes doesn't care what you like or don't like.* Whether something is good or bad for your diabetes has little to do with how much you enjoy it. My glucometer readings drove that lesson home.

A few days later, I checked my blood sugar after eating a sandwich made with whole wheat bread. I was dismayed to find that it pushed my blood sugar up more than 120 points. I was a little puzzled. The American Diabetes Association recommended whole-grain products as part of a healthy diet for diabetics. I figured I must be unusually sensitive to carbohydrates if something the Diabetes Association recommended raised my blood sugar so much. Regardless, it was apparent that if I didn't want my blood sugar shooting up that way, I needed to avoid even the whole wheat versions of bread, muffins, scones, bagels, and buns. That was disappointing, but in a way, it was also encouraging. Seeing the difference in the effect on my blood sugar between a steak and a couple of slices of bread made me realize what a powerful tool diet could be. No pill I prescribed to my patients made as much of an impact on their blood sugar as the difference I saw between those foods. These experiences sent me on a quest for a way to eat that would eliminate after-meal blood sugar surges yet be as satisfying as that steak dinner was.

Carb Science

Until the last thirty years, medical knowledge about various kinds of diets consisted largely of folk wisdom, isolated observations, and personal anecdotes. There were no large research studies comparing different diets, as there are today. In the 1970s, the National Institutes of Health started sponsoring diet studies, but not on low-carbohydrate diets. At the time, the onus was on researchers to prove the theory that low-*cholesterol* diets could prevent heart disease. No one conducted studies on low-carbohydrate diets. Scientists thought that reducing carbohydrates, by encouraging people to eat more cholesterol, would raise blood cholesterol levels and cause heart problems. It was not until the late 1990s, when it became apparent that low-cholesterol diets do not prevent heart disease or even lower blood cholesterol levels much, that researchers started conducting studies on the effects of low-carbohydrate diets. Indeed, the results of those studies turned existing notions about diet upside down.

In May 2003, the nation's most prestigious medical journal, the *New England Journal of Medicine*, published the results of two large studies comparing low-carbohydrate diets with low-fat diets. Both studies showed that cutting out starch and increasing dietary fat and cholesterol did not raise blood cholesterol levels at all, even when subjects ate all the fat and cholesterol they wanted. In fact, cutting carbohydrates improved the balance between good and bad cholesterol, the most accurate measure of heart disease risk.

These studies relieved any remaining concern I had about the effects that liberalizing my fat and cholesterol intake might have on my blood cholesterol level and allowed me to focus my dietary efforts on lowering my blood sugar. I began investigating the latest research on the effects of various carbohydrates on blood sugar. As it happened, this had recently become an area of intense interest for scientists.

For years, chemists have classified carbohydrates in two groups, *simple* and *complex*. Simple carbohydrates contain one or two sugar molecules. Complex carbohydrates consist of thousands of sugar molecules linked together in chains. According to that classification, table sugar is a simple carbohydrate, and most of the other plant products we eat—fruit, vegetables and starches—are complex carbohydrates.

Because of the large difference in size between simple and complex carbohydrate molecules, doctors figured that the body handles the two classes of carbohydrates differently. Because the digestive tract doesn't have to do much to simple carbohydrates to break them down to individual sugar molecules, doctors assumed that table sugar would get absorbed into the bloodstream faster and raise blood sugar more than complex carbohydrates, which require more disassembling by the digestive system. However, nobody systematically measured blood sugar levels in people after having them eat various carbohydrates to test how, in reality, each kind affects blood sugar.

A few years before I discovered my diabetes, researchers at the University of Toronto started measuring blood sugar levels in subjects given different foods. They did this very methodically. First, they figured out how much glucose each food eventually released into the bloodstream. They called this "available carbohydrate." Then they calculated how much of each food a person had to eat to consume fifty grams of available carbohydrate. They then gave fifty grams of available carbohydrate in the form of the food being tested to volunteers and measured blood sugar and insulin levels at regular intervals afterward.

What the researchers found surprised them. Some so-called complex carbohydrates raised blood sugar and insulin levels just as much as pure sugar did. For example, fifty grams of available carbohydrate in bread raised levels just as much as fifty grams of pure sugar. The same was true for several other complex carbohydrates, including common starches such as potatoes, rice, and corn.

That was the bad news for diabetics: a serving of bread, potatoes, or rice was as bad for your blood sugar as a pile of sugar the same size. But the research also produced some good news. Doctors had always thought that when it comes to raising blood sugar, all complex carbohydrates are the same—that it doesn't matter whether you get fifty grams of glucose from broccoli or fifty grams of glucose from bread. They figured that because both are so-called complex carbohydrates, they have the same effects on your blood sugar. "A carb is a carb," they used to say. But the Toronto researchers found wide variation among complex carbohydrates. Even if the amount of glucose that eventually went into the bloodstream was the same, some carbohydrates raised blood sugar and insulin levels more than others did. For example, fifty grams of glucose entering the bloodstream from peas raised blood sugar only half as much as fifty grams of glucose from bread. In fact, it was difficult to predict what various complex carbohydrates did to blood sugar from their carbohydrate content alone. Some raised blood sugar levels as much as pure sugar did, while others hardly raised them at all.

Scientists subsequently learned that the speed with which various foods break down to glucose and enter the bloodstream depends on a host of factors other than carbohydrate content, including fiber content, cell structure, liquidity, acidity, cellulose barriers, natural enzyme inhibitors, adhesion between molecules, particle size, and water, fat, and protein content. To tell for sure, you have to measure the effects on blood sugar directly in live human beings.

The Toronto researchers developed a scale for ranking the effects of various foods on blood sugar, which they called the *glycemic index*. It lists the amount fifty grams of available carbohydrate in each food raises blood sugar expressed as a percentage of the increase of blood sugar caused by fifty grams of available carbohydrate in white bread. For example, peas were said to have a glycemic index of 47 because fifty grams of available carbohydrate in peas raises blood sugar 47 percent as much as the same amount of available carbohydrate in white bread. Researchers have now measured the glycemic indexes of hundreds of foods in human subjects.

It didn't take long for diet book authors to start publishing lists of glycemic indexes to try to help people lose weight. This information allowed low-carbohydrate dieters to eat some foods they had been previously avoiding. But there was a problem with using the glycemic indexes as a guide to reducing carbohydrates. The amounts of food the researchers used to obtain those measurements bore little relationship to the amounts people typically eat. For example, to measure the effects of eating fifty grams of available carbohydrate in carrots, the researchers had to have subjects eat seven full-size carrots. To measure the effects of the same amount of available carbohydrate in spaghetti, they only had to have subjects eat 1¼ cups. This led to some conclusions that defy common sense. The glycemic index of carrots ended up being higher than that of spaghetti. The problem is that most folks don't eat seven full-size carrots all at once, but often eat more than 1¼ cups of spaghetti. A single carrot—a more realistic serving— hardly raises blood sugar at all, while a typical restaurant serving of spaghetti—about 2 cups—makes it skyrocket.

Actually, the researchers who developed the glycemic indexes didn't intend them to be used as a rating system for dieters. They were only trying to prove a point—that equal amounts of glucose coming from different carbohydrates could have different effects on blood sugar level and insulin secretion. Indeed, while their work generated new insights into how different foods behave in the digestive tract, to be more useful as a guide for eating, the glycemic indexes needed to take into account the amounts people typically eat. Indeed, a few years later, researchers at Harvard University combined the glycemic indexes with estimates of amounts of different foods people typically eat at one sitting to figure out how much real-life servings of various foods would raise blood sugar. They developed a more useful rating system called the *glycemic load*.

Table 3.1 lists the glycemic loads of typical servings of some common foods, along with their available-carbohydrate contents.

Table 3.1   Glycemic Loads of Common Foods

Food Item	Description	Available Carbohydrate (%)	Typical Serving	Glycemic Load (% of 1 slice of white bread)
Lab standard: 1 thin slice of white bread	30 g	47	N/A	100
Baked Goods				
Oatmeal cookie	1 medium	68	1 oz.	102
Apple muffin, sugarless	2½ in. diameter	32	2½ oz.	107
Cookie (average, all types)	1 medium	64	1 oz.	114
Croissant	1 medium	46	1½ oz.	127
Crumpet	1 medium	38	2 oz.	148
Bran muffin	2½ in. diameter	42	2 oz.	149
Pastry	Average serving	46	2 oz.	149
Chocolate cake	1 slice (4″ × 4″ × 1″)	47	3 oz.	154
Vanilla wafers	4 wafers	72	1 oz.	159
Graham cracker	1 rectangle	72	1 oz.	159
Blueberry muffin	2½ in. diameter	51	2 oz.	169
Pita bread	1 medium	57	2 oz.	189
Carrot cake	1 square (3″ × 3″ × 1½″)	56	2 oz.	199
Carrot muffin	2½ in. diameter	56	2 oz.	199
Waffle	7 in. diameter	37	2½ oz.	203
Doughnut	1 medium	49	2 oz.	205
Cupcake	2½ in. diameter	68	1½ oz.	213
Angel food cake	1 slice (4″ × 4″ × 1″)	58	2 oz.	216
English muffin	1 medium	47	2 oz.	224
Pound cake	1 slice (4″ × 4″ × 1″)	53	3 oz.	241
Corn muffin	2½ in. diameter	51	2 oz.	299
Pancake	5 in. diameter	73	2½ oz.	346
Alcoholic Beverages				
Liquor	1½ oz.		1½ oz.	<15
Red wine	6 oz. glass		6 oz.	<15

Food Item	Description	Available Carbohydrate (%)	Typical Serving	Glycemic Load (% of 1 slice of white bread)
Alcoholic Beverages *(continued)*				
White wine	6 oz. glass		6 oz.	<15
Beer	12 oz. can/bottle		12 oz.	<15
Nonalcoholic Beverages				
Tomato juice	8 oz. glass	4	8 oz.	36
Carrot juice	8 oz. glass	12	8 oz.	90
Grapefruit juice, unsweetened	8 oz. glass	9	8 oz.	100
Apple juice, unsweetened	8 oz. glass	12	8 oz.	109
Orange juice	8 oz. glass	10	8 oz.	118
Cranberry juice	8 oz. glass	12	8 oz.	145
Pineapple juice, unsweetened	8 oz. glass	14	8 oz.	145
Chocolate milk	8 oz. glass	10	8 oz.	82
Raspberry smoothie	8 oz. glass	16	8 oz.	127
Coca-Cola	12 oz. can	10	12 oz.	218
Gatorade	20 oz. bottle	6	20 oz.	273
Orange soda	12 oz. can	14	12 oz.	314
Breads and Rolls				
Tortilla (wheat)	1 medium	52	1⅜ oz.	64
Pizza crust	1 slice	22	3½ oz.	70
Tortilla (corn)	1 medium	48	1¼ oz.	87
White bread	1 slice, ½ in. thick	47	1 oz.	107
Whole-meal rye bread	½ in. slice	40	2 oz.	114
Sourdough bread	½ in. slice	47	1½ oz.	114
Oat bran bread	½ in. slice	60	1½ oz.	128
Whole wheat bread	1 slice, ½ in. thick	43	1½ oz.	129
Light rye bread	½ in. slice	47	1½ oz.	142

continues

Table 3.1 *(continued)*

Food Item	Description	Available Carbohydrate (%)	Typical Serving	Glycemic Load (% of 1 slice of white bread)
Breads and Rolls *(continued)*				
Banana bread, sugarless	1 slice (4″ × 4″ × 1″)	48	3 oz.	170
80% whole-kernel oat bread	½ in. slice	63	1½ oz.	170
Pita bread	8 in. diameter	57	2 oz.	189
Hamburger bun	5 in. diameter, top and bottom	50	2½ oz.	213
80% whole-kernel wheat bread	½ in. slice	67	2¼ oz.	213
French bread	1 slice, ½ in. thick	50	2 oz.	284
Bagel	1 medium	50	3⅓ oz.	340
Breakfast Cereals				
All-Bran	½ cup	77	1 oz.	85
Muesli	1 cup	53	1 oz.	95
Special K	1 cup	70	1 oz.	133
Cheerios	1 cup	40	1 oz.	142
Shredded wheat	1 cup	67	1 oz.	142
Grape-Nuts	1 cup	70	1 oz.	142
Puffed wheat	1 cup	70	1 oz.	151
Instant oatmeal (cooked)	1 cup	10	8 oz.	154
Cream of Wheat (cooked)	1 cup	10	8 oz.	154
Total	1 cup	73	1 oz.	161
Cornflakes	1 cup	77	1 oz.	199
Rice Krispies	1 cup	87	1 oz.	208
Rice Chex	1 cup	87	1 oz.	218
Raisin Bran	1 cup	63	2 oz.	227
Candy				
Life Saver	1 piece	100	⅒ oz.	20
Peanut M&M's	1 snack-size package	57	¾ oz.	43

Food Item	Description	Available Carbohydrate (%)	Typical Serving	Glycemic Load (% of 1 slice of white bread)
Candy *(continued)*				
White chocolate	2 squares (1″ × 1″ × ¼″)	44	⅔ oz.	49
Chocolate	2 squares (1″ × 1″ × ¼″)	44	1 oz.	68
Snickers bar	1 regular-size bar	57	2 oz.	218
Jelly beans	⅓ cup	93	1½ oz.	312
Chips and Crackers				
Potato chips	1 small bag	42	1 oz.	62
Corn chips	1 package	52	1 oz.	97
Popcorn	4 cups	55	1 oz.	114
Rye crisps	1 rectangle	64	1 oz.	125
Wheat Thins	4 small	68	1 oz.	136
Soda crackers	2 regular size	68	1 oz.	136
Pretzels	1 small bag	67	1 oz.	151
Dairy Products				
Eggs	2 eggs	0	1½ oz.	<15
Cheese	1 slice (2″ × 2″ × 1″)	0	2 oz.	<15
Butter	1 tbsp.	0	¼ oz.	<15
Margarine	1 tbsp.	0	¼ oz.	<15
Sour cream	2 tbsp.	0	2 oz.	<15
Yogurt, plain unsweetened	½ cup	5	4 oz.	17
Milk, whole	8 oz. glass	5	8 oz.	27
Yogurt, low-fat, sweetened	½ cup	16	4 oz.	57
Vanilla ice cream, high-fat	½ cup	18	4 oz.	68
Milk, low-fat chocolate	8 oz. glass	10	8 oz.	82
Vanilla ice cream, low-fat	½ cup	20	4 oz.	114

continues

Table 3.1 *(continued)*

Food Item	Description	Available Carbohydrate (%)	Typical Serving	Glycemic Load (% of 1 slice of white bread)
Dairy Products *(continued)*				
Frozen tofu	½ cup	30	4 oz.	379
Fruit				
Strawberries	1 cup	3	5½ oz.	13
Apricot	1 medium	8	2 oz.	24
Grapefruit	½ medium	9	4½ oz.	32
Plum	1 medium	10	3 oz.	36
Kiwi fruit	1 medium	10	3 oz.	43
Peach	1 medium	9	4 oz.	47
Grapes	1 cup (40 grapes)	15	2½ oz.	47
Pineapple	1 slice (¾″ thick × 3½″ diam.)	11	3 oz.	50
Watermelon, cubed	1 cup	5	5½ oz.	52
Pear	1 medium	9	6 oz.	57
Mango	½ cup	14	3 oz.	57
Orange	1 medium	9	6 oz.	71
Apple	1 medium	13	5½ oz.	78
Banana	1 medium	17	3¼ oz.	85
Raisins	2 tbsp.	73	1 oz.	133
Figs	3 medium	43	2 oz.	151
Dates	5 medium	67	1½ oz.	298
Meat				
Beef	10 oz. steak	0	10 oz.	<15
Pork	2 chops, 5 oz. each	0	10 oz.	<15
Chicken	1 breast	0	10 oz.	<15
Fish	8 oz. fillet	0	8 oz.	<15
Lamb	3 chops, 4 oz. each	0	12 oz.	<15

Food Item	Description	Available Carbohydrate (%)	Typical Serving	Glycemic Load (% of 1 slice of white bread)
Nuts				
Peanuts	¼ cup	8	1¼ oz.	7
Cashews	¼ cup	26	1¼ oz.	21
Pasta				
Asian bean noodles	2 cups	25	10 oz.	236
Whole-meal spaghetti	2 cups	23	10 oz.	252
Vermicelli	2 cups	24	10 oz.	252
Spaghetti (boiled 5 min.)	2 cups	27	10 oz.	284
Fettuccine	2 cups	23	10 oz.	284
Noodles (instant, cooked 2 min.)	2 cups	22	10 oz.	300
Capellini	2 cups	25	10 oz.	316
Spaghetti (boiled 10–15 min.)	2 cups	27	10 oz.	324
Linguine	2 cups	25	10 oz.	362
Macaroni	2 cups	28	10 oz.	362
Rice noodles	2 cups	22	10 oz.	362
Spaghetti (boiled 20 min.)	2 cups	24	10 oz.	426
Macaroni and cheese (boxed)	2 cups	28	10 oz.	504
Gnocchi	2 cups	27	10 oz.	520
Soups				
Tomato soup	1 cup	7	8 oz.	55
Minestrone	1 cup	7	8 oz.	64
Lentil soup	1 cup	8	8 oz.	82
Split pea soup	1 cup	11	8 oz.	145
Black bean soup	1 cup	11	8 oz.	154
Sweeteners				
Artificial sweeteners	1 tsp.	0	⅛ oz.	<15
Honey	1 tsp.	72	⅛ oz.	16

continues

Table 3.1 ***(continued)***

Food Item	Description	Available Carbohydrate (%)	Typical Serving	Glycemic Load (% of 1 slice of white bread)
Sweeteners *(continued)*				
Table sugar	1 round tsp.	100	⅙ oz.	28
Syrup	¼ cup	100	2 oz.	364
Vegetables				
Lettuce	1 cup	3	2½ oz.	<15
Spinach	1 cup	10	2½ oz.	<15
Cucumber	1 cup	2	6 oz.	<15
Mushrooms	½ cup	7	2 oz.	<15
Asparagus	4 spears	6	3 oz.	<15
Pepper	½ medium	6	2 oz.	<15
Broccoli	½ cup	6	1½ oz.	<15
Carrot (raw)	1 medium (7½ in. long)	10	3 oz.	11
Tomato	medium	6	5 oz.	<15
Peas	¼ cup	9	1½ oz.	16
Carrot (boiled)	½ cup	17	3 oz.	34
Kidney beans	½ cup	17	3 oz.	40
Navy beans	½ cup	10	3 oz.	40
Garbanzo beans	½ cup	20	3 oz.	45
Lima beans	½ cup	12	3 oz.	57
Pinto beans	½ cup	17	3 oz.	57
Black-eyed peas	½ cup	20	3 oz.	74
Yam	½ cup	24	5 oz.	123
Potato (instant mashed)	¾ cup	13	5 oz.	161
Sweet potato	½ cup	19	5 oz.	161
Corn on the cob	1 ear	21	5⅓ oz.	171
French fries	med. serving (McDonald's)	19	5¼ oz.	219
Baked potato	1 medium	20	5 oz.	246
Rice				
Couscous	½ cup	23	4 oz.	174
Brown rice	1 cup	22	6½ oz.	222

Food Item	Description	Available Carbohydrate (%)	Typical Serving	Glycemic Load (% of 1 slice of white bread)
Rice *(continued)*				
Basmati rice	1 cup	25	6½ oz.	271
White rice	1 cup	24	6½ oz.	283
Rice cakes	1 medium	84	1 oz.	193
Miscellaneous				
Salad dressing	typical serving		2 oz.	<15

The glycemic-load numbers reflect the percentage a typical serving raises blood sugar compared with a standard—that is, one slice of white bread. For example, a medium-sized apple has a glycemic load of 78, which means a typical serving—one apple—raises blood sugar 78 percent as much as a one-ounce slice of white bread does. Notice that a typical serving of one full-sized carrot raises blood sugar only 11 percent as much as a slice of white bread, while a restaurant serving of spaghetti raises it 324 percent.

The glycemic-load measurements painted a picture that was considerably different from the glycemic index. The impact on blood sugar of typical servings of many common grain-based carbohydrates—bread, breakfast cereals, pasta, potatoes, rice, and corn—is not just a little higher than fruits or vegetables, as the glycemic index suggests. They are *much* higher. As you can see from Table 3.1, you would have to eat seven peaches (glycemic load: 47) all at once to raise your blood sugar as much as you would by eating one bagel (glycemic load: 340). Although fresh fruits and vegetables raise blood sugar a little, they don't even come close to the effects of bread, potatoes, and rice.

Sugar Is Not the Problem

The glycemic-load measurements might have been bad news for folks who like bread, potatoes, and rice, but they were extremely good news for those of us with a sweet tooth. As it turns out, when it comes to raising blood glucose levels, sugar isn't the poison it was made out to be. Here's why.

Ounce for ounce, sugar raises blood sugar just as much bread, potatoes, or rice; that is, its glycemic *index* (not load) is just as high. For example, because Life Savers candies are mainly sugar, they have a glycemic index as high as that of bread, which means fifty grams of Life Savers consumed all at once would raise your blood sugar as much as fifty grams of bread would. However, the glycemic *load* of Life Savers is much smaller than that of bread because *the size of a typical serving of Life Savers is much smaller than the size of a typical serving of bread.* Most of us don't eat fifty grams of Life Savers—the equivalent of fifteen or twenty of them—at a time. A typical serving of Life Savers—that is, one Life Saver—is only three grams. Even though it is solid sugar, the impact on your blood sugar of one Life Saver is a fraction of that of a slice of bread—a glycemic load of 10 versus 100.

Here's another example. A person who is unaware of the glycemic loads of various foods might feel guilty about adding a teaspoon or two of sugar to a cup of coffee. Indeed, the glycemic *index* (not load) of table sugar is as high as that of baked potato—fifty grams of table sugar raises blood glucose levels as much as fifty grams of baked potato. However, you don't need a pile of sugar the size of a potato to sweeten your coffee. A teaspoon or two will do. The glycemic load of a teaspoon of sugar is only 28 compared with 256 for a typical-size baked potato.

The glycemic load of a couple of squares of dark chocolate is only 50. That was very good news to me.

A Cure for Food Cravings

For me, being able to eat a wider variety of carbohydrates was liberating. My strict low-carbohydrate regimen worked fine for keeping my blood sugar down, but truthfully, I was getting tired of it. I craved some of the foods I was avoiding, especially fruit, vegetables, milk, and sweets.

I wasn't alone. Before I learned about the glycemic load, my strict low-carb regimen was similar to the so-called Atkins diet, which had become popular at the time. In the 1960s, New York cardiologist Robert C. Atkins noticed that as long as his over-weight patients diligently avoided carbohydrates, they could eat all of the rich food they wanted and still lose weight. He developed an eating plan that sharply restricted all foods the digestive tract broke down into sugar, including sweets, starches, milk, and many fruits and vegetables. The only carbohydrates he allowed were limited amounts of green leafy vegetables. On the other hand, dieters could eat unlimited amounts of food containing fat and cholesterol, including eggs, cheese, red meat, and oils. In 1971, he published his dietary advice in a book called *The Atkins Diet Revolution.*

Atkins was far from being the first doctor to discover the potent weight-loss benefits of cutting carbs. In 1864, an over-weight British undertaker named William Banting, having failed several weight-loss schemes, consulted a prominent London physician, who recommended that he concentrate on eliminating starch and sugar. When this proved successful, Banting published a pamphlet about the diet, which was widely read in Europe and America. For almost a century, people used his name as a verb, saying they were "banting" when they were avoiding carbohydrates. In fact, reducing carbohydrates continued to be a popular way to lose weight until the 1970s, when doctors started worrying about cholesterol.

Atkins was an experienced heart specialist. He insisted that his liberalized-fat-and-cholesterol diet didn't increase the risk of heart problems or even raise blood cholesterol levels. Patients of his who lost weight seemed all the healthier for it—they felt better, their blood tests looked fine, and they didn't have any more blood vessel trouble than other people.

Unfortunately, Atkins's timing couldn't have been worse. For the first time in its history, the United States government was venturing into the realm of providing dietary advice to the public for preventing heart disease. On the basis of conclusions drawn by a handful of laypersons on a Senate committee on nutrition, government agencies started sounding alarms about cholesterol. Atkins's liberalized-fat-and-cholesterol approach to weight loss was anathema to them. He was even called before a congressional subcommittee to defend his views and was publicly derided for promoting a diet that the bureaucrats thought was harmful. As the nation fell into the grips of cholesterol paranoia, Atkins's diet quickly fell from popularity. It soon became dogma that the best way to lose weight was to reduce fat and cholesterol and eat more carbohydrates.

Twenty-five years after the government started advocating low-cholesterol diets, researchers started noticing that more and more Americans were getting fat and the rate of diabetes was rising. Despite public acceptance of the notion that dietary fat was the main cause of obesity, the low-fat approach to weight loss didn't seem to be working. It soon became obvious that the nation was experiencing an epidemic of obesity and diabetes.

By the 1990s, many people were desperate to lose weight and willing to try anything—pills, surgery, jaw wiring, whatever it took. Finally, some dieters ignored warnings about cholesterol and went back to the Atkins diet. They were pleased to find again that it worked. As long as they avoided carbohydrates, they could eat satisfying amounts of good food and still lose weight.

Doctors, for their part, were chagrined. They expected an epidemic of high blood cholesterol, but such a scourge never materialized. One difference between the 1970s and the 1990s was that in the 1990s, doctors routinely checked blood cholesterol. They also had better means of diagnosing heart disease. It became obvious that most folks who followed the Atkins diet did not develop high blood cholesterol—their blood levels of bad cholesterol usually didn't change. In fact, the balance between good and bad cholesterol—the most important risk indicator—usually *improved*. They lost weight and just seemed healthier for it.

Why did it take so long for the medical profession to realize that low carb diets don't raise blood cholesterol levels? Scientists were hesitant to conduct experiments on low-carbohydrate diets because they knew subjects would eat more fat and cholesterol, which they feared would cause heart problems. It took experts like Dr. Atkins, who had enough knowledge and experience to know that dietary cholesterol is not what causes high blood cholesterol, to eventually convince the world that low-carbohydrate diets are safe. It wasn't until the late 1990s that researchers finally began conducting carefully controlled studies on low-carbohydrate, liberalized-fat-and-cholesterol diets. They found that, indeed, such diets were more effective than low-fat diets for losing weight and did not raise blood cholesterol levels. In fact, the balance between good and bad cholesterol levels, the most accurate measurement of heart-attack risk, usually improved. It had taken thirty years for scientists to figure out that Atkins was right. Sadly, Atkins died in an accident a couple of months before the nation's leading medical journal published the results of those studies.

During the resurgence of the Atkins diet, I saw several over-weight patients who tried the program, and the results were often amazing. Their bellies would melt away even as they ate copious amounts of rich food. They felt great, and their cholesterol and blood sugar measurements looked better than ever. It was as if they had purged their bodies of a toxin that had been poisoning them for years. No wonder "banting" had been so popular for so many years. There's no doubt that it's a very effective way to shed excess fat.

The Nemesis of the Atkins Diet: Food Cravings

Just when the medical profession was beginning to appreciate the benefits of reducing carbohydrates, something interesting happened. The Atkins diet fell from popularity again. You would think that a diet that allows people to eat all of the rich food they want and produces such gratifying results would be easy to follow, but while millions of people tried Atkins's radical low-carbohydrate diet, most of them soon gave it up. The problem was food cravings. Dieters usually had no trouble following the diet at first, but typically, after a week or two, they would start yearning for the foods that were missing—fruits, vegetables, starches, milk products, and sweets. The Atkins diet fell from popularity the second time not because of cholesterol fears, not even because of hunger (remember, you could eat all you wanted). Dieters gave it up because they craved the particular foods that were missing.

So it turns out that I wasn't the only one who got tired of a strict low-carb diet. Fortunately, the glycemic load came to my rescue. New scientific insights into the effects of different carbohydrates on blood sugar put many of the foods I craved back into my diet. I found out that I didn't have to worry about most fruits and vegetables. Sure, some raise blood sugar more than others do, but none raise it nearly as much as refined carbohydrates such as baked goods, breakfast cereals, pasta, potatoes, and rice do. Although milk contains lactose, or "milk sugar," it doesn't raise blood sugar enough to worry about. I could even go back to eating a little chocolate. Learning that the blood sugar response to various foods correlates better with their glycemic loads than with their carbohydrate content—and having a list of glycemic loads to refer to—made living with diabetes much easier.

As I learned more about the glycemic load, however, I discovered that you don't need a list to tell you what foods to avoid. There are only a few culprits, and you can spot them from across the room.

4

The Culprit, Revealed

After consulting the International Table of Glycemic Index and Glycemic Load Values several times, I noticed that the serving sizes the scientists used in calculating glycemic loads were very rough approximations. Much of the data came from different countries, and the serving sizes sometimes differed significantly from the amounts Americans typically eat. For example, the researchers based their calculations for white bread on Australian slices weighing thirty grams, whereas the slices my wife brought home from the grocery store weighed forty-two grams. I decided to recalculate the glycemic loads using serving sizes that I personally verified. After a couple of weeks of prowling grocery store aisles, recording the sizes of food items and measuring typical servings at home with a scale, I compiled a more accurate list of glycemic loads for several dozen common foods.

I also noticed that the glycemic loads in the international tables were for common food *units*—for example, *slices* of bread or *cups* of pasta. Often, they didn't take into account how many such units people typically eat at one time. For example, sandwiches contain not one but two slices of bread. Restaurants usually serve not one but two cups of spaghetti, so I recalculated the values again to reflect the number of food units people typically eat.

When I put the revised list in descending order, so that the foods with the highest glycemic loads were on top and the ones with the smallest ones were on the bottom, a striking pattern emerged. As you can see in Table 4.1, *every food with a glycemic load greater than 100 was either a starch-containing solid or a sugar-containing liquid.* This actually amounted to only four kinds of food: flour products, potatoes, rice, and soft drinks. In contrast, *virtually all fresh produce—meat, dairy products, fresh fruit and vegetables—had glycemic loads less than 100.*

What was most striking about this breakdown was that the glycemic loads of the starches—baked goods, pasta, potatoes, rice, and breakfast cereals—were not just a little higher than other carbohydrates; they were *several times* higher. None of the other foods came close. For years, I had advised diabetics to limit their intake of sugar-containing fruit, such as apples and peaches, but according to my calculations, you would have to eat four apples to equal the glycemic load of a single pancake. You would have to gobble up eight peaches to match the glycemic load of a sandwich. Not even sugar or candy, the supposed nemeses of diabetics, matched the wallop delivered by starch. You would have to eat twelve teaspoons of pure sugar or ten one-inch squares of chocolate to match the glycemic load of a bagel. For years, I had listened to patients express remorse about eating a couple of pieces of chocolate or adding a teaspoon of sugar to their coffee. Rarely did they seem to worry about bread, potatoes, or rice.

Only one other kind of food—if you call it food—has glycemic loads as high as starches: sugar-containing beverages. However, most grown-ups who are the least bit concerned about diabetes or their weight know they shouldn't drink sugary soft drinks. For adults, the main problem is, indeed, the starches. According to the Nurses' Health Study, a detailed analysis of the diets of 17,000 American nurses, the combined cumulative glycemic loads of grain products, potatoes, and rice in the average woman's diet is more than twenty times that of any other food, including sugar and candy. That's the *average* consumption. The same study showed

Table 4.1 **Glycemic Loads of Common Foods in Descending Order**

Food Item	Description	Typical Serving	Glycemic Load (% of 1 slice of white bread)
Pancake	5 in. diameter	2½ oz.	346
Bagel	1 medium	3⅓ oz.	340
Orange soda	12 oz. can	12 oz.	314
Macaroni	2 cups	10 oz.	301
White rice	1 cup	6½ oz.	283
Spaghetti	2 cups	10 oz.	276
White bread	2 slices, ½ in. thick	2¾ oz.	260
Baked potato	1 medium	5 oz.	246
Whole wheat bread	2 slices, ½ in. thick	2¾ oz.	234
Raisin bran	1 cup	2 oz.	227
Brown rice	1 cup	6½ oz.	222
French fries	1 medium serving, McDonald's	5¼ oz.	219
Coca-Cola	12 oz. can	12 oz.	218
Hamburger bun	5 in. diameter, top and bottom	2½ oz.	213
English muffin	1 medium	2 oz.	208
Doughnut	1 medium	2 oz.	205
Cornflakes	1 cup	1 oz.	199
Corn on the cob	1 ear	5⅓ oz.	171
Blueberry muffin	2½ in. diameter	2 oz.	169
Instant oatmeal (cooked)	1 cup	8 oz.	154
Chocolate cake	4″ × 4″ × 1″	3 oz.	154
Grape-Nuts	1 cup	1 oz.	142
Cheerios	1 cup	1 oz.	142
Special K	1 cup	1 oz.	133
Cookie	1 medium	1 oz.	114
Lab standard: white bread	1 small slice (4″ × 4″ × ¼″)	1¹⁄₁₆ oz.	100
Tortilla, corn	1 medium	1¼ oz.	85
Banana	1 medium	3¼ oz.	85
All-Bran	½ cup	1 oz.	85
Tortilla, wheat	1 medium	1¾ oz.	80
Apple	1 medium	5½ oz.	78

continues

Table 4.1   *(continued)*

Food Item	Description	Typical Serving	Glycemic Load (% of 1 slice of white bread)
Grapefruit juice, unsweetened	6 oz. glass	6 oz.	75
Orange	1 medium	6 oz.	71
Pinto beans	½ cup	3 oz.	57
Pear	1 medium	6 oz.	57
Pineapple	1 slice (¾″ thick × 3½″ diam.)	3 oz.	50
Peach	1 medium	4 oz.	47
Grapes	1 cup (40 grapes)	2½ oz.	47
Kidney beans	½ cup	3 oz.	40
Grapefruit	½ medium	4½ oz.	32
Table sugar	1 round tsp.	⅙ oz.	28
Milk (whole)	8 oz. glass	8 oz.	27
Peas	¼ cup	1½ oz.	16
Tomato	1 medium	5 oz.	15
Strawberries	1 cup	5½ oz.	13
Carrot (raw)	1 medium (7½ in. length)	3 oz.	11
Peanuts	¼ cup	1¼ oz.	7
Spinach	1 cup	2½ oz.	0
Pork	2 chops (5 oz. each)	10 oz.	0
Margarine	1 tbsp.	¼ oz.	0
Lettuce	1 cup	2½ oz.	0
Fish	8 oz. fillet	8 oz.	0
Eggs	2 eggs	1½ oz.	0
Cucumber	1 cup	6 oz.	0
Chicken	1 breast	10 oz.	0
Cheese	1 slice (2″ × 2″ × 1″)	2 oz.	0
Butter	1 tbsp.	¼ oz.	0
Broccoli	½ cup	1½ oz.	0
Beef	10 oz. steak	10 oz.	0

Table 4.2   **Low-Glycemic-Load Versus Typical Eating Pattern**

Low-Glycemic-Load Pattern		Glycemic Load	Typical Pattern		Glycemic Load
Breakfast	Bacon	32	**Breakfast**	Orange juice	68
	Eggs	0		Bagel	340
	Coffee, 1 tsp.			Coffee (black)	0
	sugar	28			
Snack	Latte	27	**Snack**	Coffee	0
	Apple	78		Doughnut	205
Lunch	Chicken Caesar	0	**Lunch**	Turkey sandwich	260
	salad (no croutons)			Potato chips	77
	Milk	27		Coca-Cola	218
Snack	Mixed nuts	7	**Snack**	Corn chips	97
Dinner	Green salad	0	**Dinner**	Caesar salad (with	
	Large steak	0		croutons)	100
	Mushrooms	0		Spaghetti, 2 cups	276
	Asparagus	0		French bread	284
	1/3 baked potato	82		Butter	0
	Butter	0		Red wine	0
	Sour cream	0			
	Red wine	0			
Dessert	Dark chocolate	68	**Dessert**	Cookie	114
Total Glycemic Load:		**349**	**Total Glycemic Load:**		**2,043**

that women who developed diabetes ate significantly *more* than average amounts of starch.

If you have trouble believing that a few starchy foods can have such a big effect on your body's demands for insulin, look at Table 4.2, which tallies up the daily glycemic load in the typical diet of a person not trying to limit refined carbohydrates compared with the diet of a person who avoids them. As you can see, a day's total glycemic load—and thus the body's demands for insulin—for a person consuming typical amounts of starch and sugar-containing beverages can easily end up being five or six times that of a person eating just as heartily but avoiding a few starchy foods. Notice that you can put sugar in your coffee, have some chocolate after dinner, and still keep your glycemic load much lower than it would be if you ate typical amounts of starch and sugar-containing beverages.

The Great American Cholesterol Experiment

In the 1970s, government agencies and professional organizations began telling Americans to limit their intake of fat and cholesterol and not worry much about flour products, potatoes, and rice. However, once I learned about the glycemic load and saw the effects refined carbohydrates had on my after-meal blood sugar readings, I started to wonder what effects America's thirty-year fixation on avoiding fat and cholesterol and relative lack of concern about carbohydrates was having on the incidence of diabetes and obesity. So I did some fact-finding on my own.

I was skeptical of things I had heard or read about diet. Health gurus, vegetarians, animal rights advocates, and commercial interests all have strong views about what people should or should not eat, and they don't seem to be hesitant to express them. However, their opinions usually lack solid scientific proof. I could see that when it comes to diet, bias creeps into the recommendations made by even reputable scientific organizations.

One problem is that carefully controlled studies on diet are difficult to conduct. You can't put people in pens and control what they eat as you can laboratory animals. However, if you think about it, we all live in a sort of pen—the one defined by our national borders. Since the 1940s, the United States Department of Agriculture (USDA) has kept detailed records of the nation's consumption of different foods. In the 1960s, the National Health Assessment and Nutrition Examination Survey (NHANES) started monitoring the incidences of obesity and diabetes. If you combine these two sources of data, you come up with some enlightening facts.

For years now, we Americans have been told by government agencies, vegetarian groups, and animal rights advocates that we eat too much fat and cholesterol, the main sources being red meat, eggs, and fatty dairy products. However, according to USDA data, consumption of these foods has been steadily *declining* since the

Table 4.3 **Yearly Consumption per Person of Red Meat, Eggs, and Milk Fat, 1970 Versus 1997**

Type of Food	1970	1997	Change from 1970 to 1997
Red meat	132 lb.	111 lb.	Down 16%
Eggs	309 eggs	239 eggs	Down 23%
Milk fat (equivalent in whole milk)	114 qt.	55 qt.	Down 52%

early 1960s. As you can see in Table 4.3, by 1997, Americans were consuming 16 percent less red meat, 23 percent fewer eggs, and 52 percent less milk fat per person than they did in 1970.

That surprised me at first, but the more I thought about it, the more obvious it was. I was practicing medicine then. I saw that people actually were trying to reduce their consumption of fat and cholesterol. They had been convinced that cholesterol-containing foods raise blood cholesterol levels, and that dietary fat is the main cause of obesity. Vegetarianism had become popular, and animal-rights advocates and environmentalists were reminding us that eating animal products is unkind to other species and hard on the planet. In addition, in the 1970s, inflation pushed up prices of eggs, meat, and dairy products relative to other foods.

So what were the results of this nationwide shift away from fat and cholesterol? It had little effect on the incidence of heart disease, but it triggered an epidemic of obesity and diabetes. By 1997, the percentage of obese Americans doubled, and the diabetes rate tripled. What happened?

There's nothing inherently wrong with cutting back on eggs, meat, and dairy products. The problem is that if you eat less of one kind of food, you invariably eat more of another. As you might predict, when Americans started reducing their consumption of fat and cholesterol, they began eating more carbohydrates—but not carbohydrates in their natural state, like fresh fruit and veg-etables. They started eating more processed carbs—flour products, frozen potato products (read french fries), and rice—and not just a little more, a *lot* more. As you can see in Table 4.4, by 1997, Americans were consuming 48 percent more wheat products, 186

Table 4.4   **Yearly Consumption per Person of Wheat Flour, Rice, and Frozen Potato Products, 1970 Versus 1997**

Type of Food	1970	1997	Change from 1970 to 1997
Flour	135 lb.	200 lb.	Up 48%
Rice	7 lb.	20 lb.	Up 186%
Frozen potato products (mainly french fries)	13 lb.	30 lb.	Up 131%

percent more rice, and 131 percent more frozen potato products per person than they did in 1970.

The largest source of carbohydrate in the American diet by far is our old friend from the Fertile Crescent, wheat—the food that kicked off the Agricultural Revolution. We eat it in the form of bread, bagels, pasta, breakfast cereals, buns, muffins, and more. To illustrate how rising wheat consumption correlates with rising obesity, the graph in Figure 4.1 compares the average wheat consumption per person between 1961 and 2000 with the percentage of the population who were thirty pounds or more overweight. You can see that in the 1970s, wheat consumption started rising sharply, and shortly afterward, the obesity rate, which correlates with the diabetes rate, rose in perfect tandem.

What about sugar? Because diabetes causes high blood glucose, which is a type of sugar, many diabetics conclude, incorrectly, that dietary sugar, such as in candy and table sugar, is the main problem. Indeed, by 1997 Americans were consuming 26 percent more sugar than they did in 1970. However, this was not in the form of candy or table sugar. The consumption of these sweets stayed the same. The increase came from kids consuming more sugar in the form of soft drinks and adults consuming more in sweetened flour products such as cookies, snack bars, and pastries.

Despite the fact that fat and cholesterol consumption in the United States has declined steadily for thirty years, we Americans are still told that we're eating too much fat and cholesterol. We have been led to believe that to get fat, you have to eat fat and that the cholesterol in your blood comes from cholesterol in food. Most

Figure 4.1 **Obesity Rate Versus Annual Wheat Consumption per Person (1961–2000)**

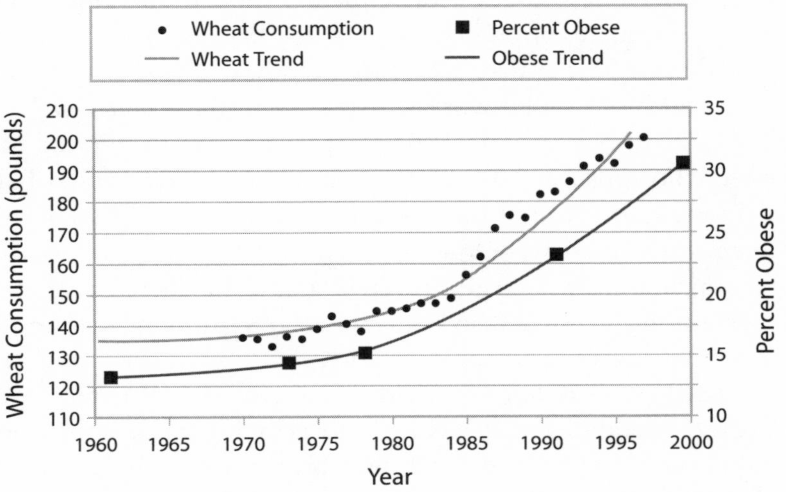

Source: National Center for Health Statistics Third National Health and Nutrition Examination Survey and U.S. Department of Agriculture National Nutrient Database

people don't realize—and many doctors seem to have forgotten—that the body can turn carbohydrates into fat within minutes and the body makes its own cholesterol. The brown rice you had for dinner last night? By now some of it has turned into the same kind of fat and cholesterol you've been told for years you should avoid.

It might seem a curious coincidence that the three foods that dominate the top of the glycemic-load list—wheat products, potatoes, and rice—are the same three foods Americans suddenly began eating more of starting in the 1970s. It's almost as though folks looked at the glycemic-load list and started *trying* to eat more high-glycemic-load foods. This is no accident. In later chapters, you will see that the unique chemical and biological properties that cause these foods to raise blood sugar also created cultural and economic forces that have caused humans to eat increasing amounts of them.

The fact that for thirty years the incidence of diabetes and obesity has closely paralleled rising starch consumption suggests that excessive consumption of refined carbohydrates does more than cause trouble for people who already have diabetes. It brings on the disease in the first place. In a study of the effects of diet on the health of 85,059 women, reported in the *American Journal of Clinical Nutrition* in 2008, Harvard researchers found that women who consumed diets high in starch had a two-and-a-half-fold increase in the risk of developing diabetes compared with women whose diets were low in starch. The increased risk of diabetes was not just the result of weight gain. The diabetes rate was higher among women who consumed large amounts of starch, whether they were overweight or not.

Actually, this is not surprising. Diabetes is a disease of carbohydrate metabolism. It has little to do with fat or cholesterol metabolism. Your body doesn't need insulin to metabolize fat or cholesterol, only carbohydrates. Excessive demands for insulin can occur only when carbohydrate intake is excessive.

Starch Diabetes

The most common barrier to good control of blood sugar is improper diet. You can take all the drugs your doctor has to offer, but if you don't get your diet right, you're unlikely to get a good handle on your blood sugar. You might get your fasting levels down, but unless you reduce the glycemic load of your diet, you'll repeatedly flood your bloodstream with glucose and increase your risk of eye, kidney, and blood-vessel damage.

Many diabetic patients I meet for the first time don't realize which foods raise their blood sugar. Because doctors often say blood "sugar" when they mean blood *glucose,* it's understandable that patients think the problem is sugar—that is, the kind you put in your coffee. Some folks still call diabetes "sugar diabetes." Make no mistake, dietary sugar is *not* what usually raises blood sugar. The culprit is starch—baked goods, potatoes, pasta, rice, breakfast cereals, and so on. Starch is not just the worst offender; for practical purposes, *it's the only offender.* A better name than sugar diabetes would be starch diabetes!

Hung Up on Cholesterol, Blindsided by Starch

No longer is the relationship between starch and diabetes difficult to see. Scientists have pointed it out numerous times, but until lately, government agencies and medical organizations downplayed it. As the diabetes and obesity rates continued to climb, they kept telling diabetics not to worry about starch, but just to avoid fat and cholesterol. Given that starch is virtually the worst thing you can eat if you want to control your blood sugar, the diet that doctors recommended for diabetics was better in the 1890s than it was in the 1990s. How did the medical profession get so far off track?

Before diabetes pills became available in the 1950s, the only way adult-onset diabetics could control their blood sugar without taking insulin shots was, indeed, to avoid foods the digestive system turns to sugar. Nobody worried about cholesterol. Most folks hadn't even heard of it. In the 1960s, scientists discovered links between high blood levels of cholesterol and heart disease and made an assumption that changed doctors' recommendations to diabetics. Doctors assumed—*incorrectly*—that high levels of cholesterol in the blood come from eating too much cholesterol. Because diabetes causes blood-vessel problems, doctors thought diabetics would be especially likely to benefit from reducing cholesterol consumption. Consequently, they began advising diabetics to reduce their consumption of cholesterol-containing foods.

The experts at the time knew that reducing cholesterol would have no effect on blood sugar levels—the systems in the body that deal with cholesterol are largely separate from the ones that regulate blood sugar. However, they figured that avoiding dietary cholesterol would help control blood sugar in an indirect way. Because most cholesterol-containing foods contain fat, the experts also figured that avoiding cholesterol and the fat that goes with it would promote weight loss, and losing weight indeed makes diabetes easier to control. Doctors realized that if folks tried to cut out fat and cholesterol at the same time they tried to eliminate carbohydrates, they would run out of things to eat, so they started telling adult-onset diabetics not to worry about carbohydrates. They figured patients could use the new diabetes pills that pharmaceutical companies were promoting to lower their blood sugar. They could then focus their efforts on reducing fat and cholesterol.

By the mid-1970s, with paranoia about cholesterol on the rise, the advice to reduce dietary fat and cholesterol replaced the time-honored approach of avoiding carbohydrates. The only carbohydrate diabetics were told to avoid was sugar. The rationale was that whereas digestive enzymes had to work on other carbohydrates to break them down to glucose before they could be absorbed, sugar went directly into the bloodstream. Moreover, sugar had a bad reputation because it causes tooth decay.

Although this low-fat, high-carbohydrate, pill-taking approach to diabetes seemed logical at the time, it was based on the theory that reducing dietary fat and cholesterol could prevent heart disease. However, no one had ever proved that avoiding dietary cholesterol even lowers blood cholesterol, let alone prevents blood vessel disease. The notion that high blood cholesterol comes from eating too much fat and cholesterol seemed reasonable, but the evidence that supported it was flimsy. Researchers cited reduced rates of heart disease in certain countries whose citizens were too poor to eat much fat and cholesterol, at the same time ignoring countries with similar diets whose residents had higher rates. They also cited experiments in which scientists caused cholesterol buildup in the arteries of rabbits by feeding them fat and cholesterol, which, of course, rabbits don't normally eat.

It took years for researchers to test the theory that low-fat, low-cholesterol diets prevent heart disease. The results were disappointing. After thirty years, researchers learned that low-fat, low-cholesterol diets don't prevent heart attacks or even lower blood cholesterol levels much. Several studies showed that low-fat, low-cholesterol diets, even when supervised by professional dietitians, reduced cholesterol levels at best by only 5 to 10 percent—not enough to make much of a dent in a person's risk of blood vessel problems. To put that in perspective, modern cholesterol-lowering medications reduce levels by 50 or 60 percent, which significantly reduces the risk of heart attacks and strokes.

In 2006, researchers released the results of the Women's Health Initiative Dietary Modification Trial, a study designed to settle the question of whether low-cholesterol diets work. It was the largest, most rigorous study to investigate the effects of low-fat, low-cholesterol diets on the risk of heart and blood vessel disease. Scientists randomly assigned a total of 48,835 women to either receive intensive low-fat, low-cholesterol dietary counseling by certified nutritionists or get no counseling. The 19,541 who got the training attended eighteen low-cholesterol diet-training sessions the first year and one session every three months thereafter for eight years. Although the group that received the counseling succeeded in lowering their fat and cholesterol intake significantly, their efforts were for naught. After eight years, their average cholesterol level fell less than 2 percent, and there was no difference whatsoever in their heart attack or stroke rates.

One of the problems is that folks tend to take the old adage "You are what you eat" too literally. They figure you get fat from eating fat and get high blood cholesterol from eating cholesterol; but it doesn't work that way. Most of the cholesterol in your blood does *not* come from food. Your liver produces it. Your liver makes about three times more cholesterol than you eat. If you eat more cholesterol, it just makes less. If you eat less cholesterol, it makes more. Cholesterol is a vital substance. Your body needs it to make important things like cell membranes and hormones. Humans wouldn't have survived if they had to rely on the vicissitudes of dietary intake to provide a steady supply to the tissues that need it.

Actually, the digestive system has difficulty absorbing the cholesterol in food. Most of it passes right through your intestinal tract and out in your stool. The level of cholesterol in your blood has little to do with how much cholesterol you eat. It depends mainly on how readily your body gets rid of it, which is largely a genetic characteristic. When it comes to cholesterol, who your parents are is much more important than what you eat.

Why the myth persists that low-fat, low-cholesterol diets prevent heart disease or even lower blood cholesterol levels is curious. In 2008, the *Journal of Clinical Lipidology* published a review of *thirty* studies comparing low-fat with liberalized-fat diets. Lower fat intake had no effect on levels of bad cholesterol and actually worsened the balance between good and bad cholesterol, the most accurate predictor of heart disease. This was particularly true for diabetic patients.

In the face of overwhelming evidence that low-fat, low-cholesterol diets don't work for losing weight, lowering blood cholesterol levels, or treating diabetes and that they encourage people to eat more starch, which *is* proven harmful, some doctors, academes, bureaucrats, animal rights advocates, and environmentalists still scold folks for eating fat and cholesterol. Perhaps the reason many people are resistant to changing their ideas about diet is because they personally try to abide by the dietary patterns they advocate. Changing their ideas would require them to face the fact that their own dietary habits have been misguided.

There's also an element of political correctness in avoiding fat and cholesterol. Some social critics have hypothesized that diet has become the new morality—that a Victorian kind of food ethic has taken the place of old-style sexual morality. Morality usually involves a struggle against natural urges, and as the failure of low-fat diets has proven, abstaining from fat and cholesterol is truly a struggle against natural urges—one, in fact, that most of us lose.

As for the liberalized-carbohydrate, pill-taking approach to treating diabetes, no one succeeded in proving that the 1950s-era diabetes pills were as effective as low-carbohydrate diets for treating diabetes. Just as it took years for researchers to learn that low-cholesterol diets don't work, it took decades for doctors to figure out that just telling patients to take the pills and not bother cutting out carbohydrates didn't help them control their blood sugar very well. The pills would work OK at first, but after a year or so, they lost much of their effectiveness. They helped keep the blood sugar from rising high enough to cause dehydration but didn't reduce it enough to prevent blood vessel damage. The reason it took twenty years for researchers to learn this was that such damage often takes years to become manifest.

For several years after I started practicing medicine, I dispensed the standard advice to diabetics to reduce fat and cholesterol, take their pills, and not worry much about carbohydrates except for sweets. I sent patients to dietitians to teach them to follow the

American Diabetes Association guidelines, but it didn't seem to help much. I had lost faith in the Diabetes Association's dietary recommendations even before I got diabetes. When I got diabetes, I chose to ignore the Diabetes Association's recommendations from the start. Instead, I took the low-starch approach to treating my diabetes—and it has worked fine for ten years.

A Diet You Actually Can Follow

Every working day of my life, I counsel people about their diet—not only for diabetes but also high blood cholesterol, high blood pressure, and obesity. If there's one lesson I've learned in three decades of practicing preventive cardiology, it's that dietary habits are hard to change. People think they can change more than they can. When they fall short, they get discouraged and quit trying altogether. But eliminating starch is different. It's much easier to do than cutting calories or reducing fat, because it's not about going hungry or avoiding foods you naturally crave. It's something most people can do and continue doing for life.

For years now, I have encouraged patients with type 2 diabetes to stop worrying about fat and cholesterol, not fret over a little sugar, forget about salt, put trans fats out of their minds, and don't try to cut calories—just concentrate on eliminating starch. Among my patients who take insulin, it's unusual for those who follow a low-glycemic-load eating pattern to require more than a third of the insulin needed by those who consume typical amounts of starch. As a bonus, they usually lose weight. Indeed, the most effective weight loss programs reported in the medical literature are among patients with type 2 diabetes or prediabetes who follow a low-starch diet. In a study reported in the journal *Nutrition and Metabolism* in 2006, researchers compared a group of patients with type 2 diabetes who had been instructed to eliminate carbohydrates with a group of diabetics who were told to continue eating their usual amounts. The patients who eliminated carbohydrates required less than a third of the insulin medication needed by those who continued eating their usual amounts. Some were able to discontinue insulin altogether. After a year, they lost an average of eighteen pounds, and unlike the results of most diets reported in the medical literature, they hadn't regained the weight when the study ended twenty-two months later. In recent years, several studies reported in the medical literature have confirmed the beneficial effects experienced by patients with adult-onset diabetes and prediabetes who eliminate dietary starch.

If You're Taking Cholesterol-Lowering Medication

It's true that high blood cholesterol can be especially harmful to your blood vessels if you have diabetes, which is why many people with diabetes take cholesterol-lowering medication. Indeed, the American Diabetes Association and the American College of Cardiology recommend that most people with diabetes take cholesterol medication. Of course, this does not mean that *eating* cholesterol is hard on your blood vessels. As discussed earlier in this chapter, your blood cholesterol level is not a matter of how much cholesterol you eat; rather, it's a matter of how much your body gets rid of, and that's mainly a genetic thing. Thankfully, modern cholesterol medication can dependably correct the biochemical quirk that causes high blood cholesterol.

The most effective cholesterol-lowering medicine is a type of drug called *statins*. These include lovastatin (trade name Mevacor), pravastatin (Pravachol), simvastatin (Zocor), fluvastatin (Lescol), atorvastatin (Lipitor), and rosuvastatin (Crestor). If you're taking a statin and avoid starch, your blood cholesterol level will probably stay down, *no matter how much fat and cholesterol you eat—within reason.* In one study reported in the journal *Mayo Clinic Proceedings* in 2003, researchers fed subjects who were taking statins an astounding pound and a half of red meat and two to four eggs per day for six weeks. Their bad-cholesterol levels didn't budge. Using an advanced technique called nuclear magnetic resonance, they found that the higher fat intake caused cholesterol particles to become less dense, a quality associated with *reduced* risk of blood vessel damage.

Actually, once you get your cholesterol down with a statin, your risk of heart attack becomes more dependent on your good-cholesterol and triglyceride levels than on your bad-cholesterol level. Dozens of studies have shown that reducing dietary starch lowers triglyceride and raises good-cholesterol levels. While a low-starch diet complements statins, statins in turn complement a low-starch diet. By relieving any hang-ups you might have about eating fat and cholesterol, cholesterol-lowering medication lets you focus on eliminating starch.

5

The Highly Peculiar Effects of Dietary Starch

So what exactly is starch, and why is it so bad for you? The answer lies in starch's unique chemical structure. The building block of all plant life is the sugar glucose. Through the process of *photosynthesis*, plants manufacture glucose literally out of thin air by combining carbon dioxide in the air with water using energy from sunlight. Plant enzymes then link the glucose molecules together to form larger molecules called carbohydrates, which form the substance of plants, including the wood, leaves, roots, and fruit.

Although your body can use glucose as a source of calories, you can't just walk up to a shrub or a tree, start eating it, and expect to get any calories from it. Even if you could chew and swallow a leaf or a piece of stalk, your intestines wouldn't be able to digest it. Intestinal enzymes must break carbohydrates down to their individual glucose molecules before they can be absorbed into your bloodstream. The glucose molecules in most parts of plants and trees are linked together by strong connections, called *beta bonds*, which the human digestive system is incapable of breaking. Indeed, the vegetable kingdom is remarkably stingy when it comes to providing nutrition to humans. Of the thousands of different plant species, we're able to use only a tiny fraction for food.

However, one plant substance humans *can* digest easily is starch, which is found in high concentrations in seeds. The glucose molecules in starch are linked by much weaker connections called *alpha bonds*, which are actually made to be broken. Enzymes in seeds can break these bonds and release the glucose, which provides a readily available source of energy for seeds to grow into sprouts.

Although Mother Nature originally intended that starch be used as a source of energy for plants, not animals, the digestive enzymes of many animals are also capable of breaking the weak bonds that hold together its glucose molecules and using it for food. This is why Mother Nature encased the starch in tough husks impermeable to most predators. Only since humans developed the means to extract the cores of wheat from their husks has starch been a significant part of the human diet.

Starch Crystals

Starch is the same tasteless paste that launderers use to stiffen shirt collars. The word *starch* comes from the Old English word *sterchen*, meaning "to stiffen." The glucose in starch makes its molecules sticky when it's mixed with water, so it clings to cloth fibers. When it dries, it hardens and stiffens the fabric—not unlike what it does to your arteries.

Although the starch in seeds is powdery, each granule is actually a crystal—a tiny stone. The molecules in these rocks fit together so compactly that no other food can match starch when it comes to packing calories into a small space. As long as these crystals stay dry, they maintain their rocklike compactness and resist digestion by plant or animal enzymes. Resistance to bacterial enzymes allows starch to be stored for long periods without rotting as long as it is kept dry.

Although starch crystals are like little rocks when they're dry, they behave like sponges when wet. In the liquid environment of the digestive tract, they quickly soak up water, soften, and swell. Digestive enzymes are then able to get between the starch chains, break the bonds that hold the glucose molecules together, and free up the glucose. Starch breaks down to glucose so readily that even carnivores, whose digestive systems weren't designed to handle carbohydrates, are able to digest it. Dog and cat food manufacturers put wheat, rice, and corn in their products to save on meat, a practice that has triggered an epidemic of obesity and diabetes among pets. Indeed, diabetes in cats can be cured by allowing them to return to their natural all-meat diet.

The high concentration of glucose in starch crystals is something to keep in mind when you hear that whole-grain foods are good for you. It's true that you get more fiber in whole-grain products than in the white versions, but you also get more glucose. Those seeds are packed with crystalline starch, but unlike seeds in nature, they have been cracked open so your digestive enzymes can get to the starch. Make no mistake, whole-grain bread and brown rice can raise your blood sugar just as much as the white versions do, and they contain more calories to boot. They might be good for you if you are deficient of vitamins, but that's rarely a problem for Americans and Europeans. As for fiber, whole-grain bread and brown rice don't contain enough to do you much good.

Glucose Shocks

When you eat natural carbohydrates like fresh fruit or vegetables, glucose trickles into your bloodstream slowly over several hours. Much of the carbohydrate never gets digested and arrives in your colon as indigestible fiber. Starch behaves differently. Those tiny crystals are glucose bombs. Within minutes of hitting your intestines, they dissolve like snowballs in water, releasing pure glucose into your bloodstream. No other food, with the exception of pure sugar, delivers as much sugar into your system as fast as starch does.

Because starch puts so much glucose into your bloodstream so fast, your body needs more insulin to handle it than it does for other foods, *even if the amount of glucose that ultimately enters your bloodstream is the same*. That's the principle behind the glycemic index and load. For example, if you ate enough broccoli to supply as much glucose as a slice of bread, you would still need more insulin to handle the bread. Your body's insulin response to eating starch is like a fire department's response to a fire. If the fire is just smoldering, you only need a few firefighters to put it out. If it bursts into flames, you need a whole crew.

The glucose in fresh fruits and vegetables enters your bloodstream gradually so that your insulin-making cells can fine-tune their response. You get just the right amount of insulin at just the right time. But when you eat starch, your body requires so much more insulin to handle the glucose released that those cells have trouble fine-tuning their response. Insulin secretion often overshoots and causes the blood sugar to fall too fast. Low blood sugar, or *hypoglycemia*, causes fatigue, poor concentration, and compelling hunger, all of which are promptly relieved by eating more starch. Indeed, hypoglycemia makes people crave refined carbohydrates. Researchers at the Royal Infirmary of Edinburgh (in Scotland) gave subjects insulin to lower their blood sugar below normal levels and observed the types of foods they chose to eat. Sure enough, low blood sugar gave them a preference for starchy foods.

Beta-Cell Burnout

Because modern humans eat so much starch, they have to produce several times more insulin than their prehistoric ancestors did. However, our Stone Age insulin-making equipment wasn't designed to produce so much insulin. After years of excessive insulin production, beta cells can virtually wear out from overwork.

Beta-cell "burnout" is actually a curious phenomenon. Most cells of the body don't wear out from doing what they're supposed to do. They usually get stronger. However, when beta cells make insulin, they spin off a by-product called amylin. In small amounts, amylin is harmless; the beta cells are able to dispose of it. However, in high concentrations, its molecules stick together and form a kind of sludge, which damages the cells that produce it.

As you develop diabetes, your insulin-secreting cells start dropping out years before your fasting blood sugar levels rise. During this "prediabetic" phase, you make enough insulin to keep your blood sugar down between meals but often not enough to prevent it from rising to higher-than-normal levels after eating carbohydrates. Doctors call this "glucose intolerance." It can be diagnosed by checking your blood sugar after you eat a starchy meal. A level of 140 or higher two hours after a meal is a sign of prediabetes.

Glucose intolerance goes on for years before your *fasting* blood sugar rises, which is when doctors make diagnosis of diabetes. By that time, your beta cells have typically lost about half of their ability to produce insulin. Most of that lost capacity can never be recovered.

Excessive after-meal surges in blood sugar aren't just a sign of problems to come. These "glucose shocks" can damage blood vessels even if your blood sugar levels between meals are normal. While doctors have good medications for lowering *fasting* blood sugar, medical science hasn't come up with drugs nearly as good at reducing *after-meal* surges. You can lower the after-meal spikes by injecting rapid-acting insulin before eating, but because after-meal blood sugars are often unpredictable, the dose of insulin often falls short and fails to blunt the spike or overshoots and causes the blood sugar to fall too much. Many doctors tell their patients to not even try controlling postprandial spikes. They suggest not bothering to check blood sugar levels after meals.

There is one sure way to eliminate after-meal blood sugar surges: *Don't eat things that raise your blood sugar in the first place.* If you avoid foods with high glycemic loads—starch-containing solids and sugar-containing liquids—your blood sugar won't shoot up after eating, and you will need much less insulin.

Your Fatty Tumor

Your fat is like the gas tank in a car. It's where your body stores fuel. If you're overweight, you have a couple of months' worth of calories stored up in your fat depots.

With all those calories stored up as fat, you might wonder why an overweight person would have to eat every few hours to keep him- or herself from getting hungry. Why doesn't the body get the energy it needs from the calories stored up in fat? Here's why.

Although small amounts of insulin actually suppress appetite and encourage weight loss, in large amounts insulin becomes a potent calorie-storing hormone. It pushes calories out of your bloodstream into your fat cells. Continuously high levels of insulin hold calories in your fat deposits so your body can't get at them so that within three or four hours of eating, you're ravenous again. Your fat starts acting like a big tumor robbing you of calories as it grows. Scientists call this *internal starvation.*

When your insulin levels are as low as nature intended them to be, your body has no trouble mobilizing fat for fuel. Calories go into your fat when you eat and flow out between meals. The main cause of excessive insulin excretion is excessive starch consumption. If you eliminate starch, your insulin levels stay down, and you shed excess fat. That's why low-carbohydrate diets work so well for losing weight.

Twenty Feet of Empty Gut

You have about twenty-two feet of intestine. The reason it's so long is that it takes time for your digestive enzymes to break down and absorb most foods. As food travels the length of your intestine, your digestive enzymes have time to process it. Starch, however, has a peculiar digestive pattern. It is completely absorbed in the first foot or two of your intestine. It never reaches the other twenty feet. Indeed, if you ate nothing but starch, you would only need a couple of feet of intestine.

Doctors take advantage of starch's peculiar digestive properties when they treat certain medical conditions. Sometimes surgeons have to remove large amounts of intestine because of wounds or disease. Afterward, patients who have had such surgery sometimes can't absorb enough nutrients to sustain themselves, and they have to be fed fat, protein, and vitamins intravenously. But one thing they don't have to be fed intravenously is carbohydrate. As long as they have a couple of feet of intestine, they can digest starch just fine. So remember, starch is a great food if you've had 90 percent of your intestines removed!

If starch's digestive pattern sounds strange, that's because it is. The short-circuiting of food into your bloodstream in the first couple of feet of your intestine is unnatural. It upsets important weight-regulating mechanisms. Your digestive tract has systems in place for controlling how much food you eat. Specifically, when food gets to the last part of your intestine, specialized cells in the walls of the intestine secrete hormones that slow stomach emptying and tell your brain to stop eating. Scientists call this the "intestinal brake," because it puts the brakes on digestion. However, starch never reaches the last part of your digestive tract where those appetite-suppressing hormones are released—another reason why, a couple of hours after eating a starchy meal, you're hungry again.

In one experiment reported in the *Journal of Pediatrics* in 1999, Harvard researchers gave subjects starchy breakfasts in the form of instant oatmeal and compared their food intake for the rest of the day with that of subjects given an equal number of calories in the form of a low-glycemic-load breakfast of eggs and fresh fruit. Over a period of six weeks, the subjects who ate the starchy breakfasts consumed on average 145 more calories per day than those who ate the low-glycemic breakfasts. That's enough calories to put on sixty pounds in five years.

In addition to regulating weight, intestinal hormones also help control blood sugar. One of these, called incretin, is actually available as an injectable diabetes medication called exenatide (trade name Byetta). Not only does it help lower blood sugar in type 2 diabetics, it reliably produces weight loss.

Carbs Without Fiber

For millions of years, humans ate copious amounts of difficult-to-digest plant parts, such as grasses, bark, roots, and unripe fruit and berries. Whatever nutrition they got from plants came with plenty of indigestible carbohydrate, or "fiber," whose glucose molecules were linked by unbreakable beta bonds. The human digestive tract evolved over hundreds of thousands of years to handle a diet that contains large amounts of fiber. Indeed, our Stone Age intestinal tract functions best when we eat plenty of indigestible carbohydrate.

Fiber acts like a sponge in your intestinal tract. It soaks up nutrients and slows the absorption of glucose into your bloodstream. It also provides bulk to food as it moves through your digestive tract. Fiber is also essential for normal colon function. Inadequate intake leads to constipation, irritable bowel syndrome, diverticulosis, hemorrhoids, and other bowel problems.

Since prehistoric times, most of the fiber has been refined out of the human diet. Most of the carbohydrates people eat these days is in the form of starch, which contains virtually no fiber. In industrialized countries, lack of fiber is the most common dietary deficiency.

Tasteless Calories

If you ask people why they eat starches, they will probably tell you they enjoy the taste. This is interesting because starch is essentially flavorless. Your taste buds can't detect starch. If you don't believe that, try eating a spoonful of flour. Enzymes in your saliva break down about 2 percent of the starch you eat to sugar, which you can taste, but the rest of it ends up in your stomach without interacting with your taste buds. Ironically, while starch releases more sugar into your bloodstream than any other kind of food, you can't taste it.

So what's the harm in not tasting the sugar in starch? Scientists have found that sugar you taste satisfies your appetite more than sugar you don't taste. In one experiment, researchers infused sugar through tubes inserted into people's stomachs and compared their eating behavior afterward with that of people fed sugar orally. The subjects who were able to taste the sugar that went into their bloodstream consumed less food afterward than those who didn't.

If you can't taste starch, then what *do* you taste when you eat bread, potatoes, and rice? Well, starch soaks up substances you *can* smell and taste. When you chew it, it releases compounds interspersed among its molecules, which produce recognizable flavor overtones. Humans wouldn't like the taste of flour products, potatoes, and rice as much as they do if they couldn't add things like butter, oil, salt, sugar, spices, sauces, glazes, and jams to them.

Unless you're starving, you don't eat just anything that supplies calories; the flavor of a food affects your appetite for it. So here's the good news: because starch provides no flavor, when you remove it from your diet, you don't actually remove any flavor. In fact, if you replace it with other foods, you end up *increasing* the amount of flavor in your diet. The increase in taste bud stimulation you get by replacing starch with other foods is one reason people find it easier to stick to low-starch diets than to other kinds of diets. Research studies have repeatedly shown that people on low-starch diets who do not consciously try to reduce calories still end up consuming fewer calories than people on low-fat diets who try to cut calories.

No Survival Benefit

Mother Nature's reason for giving you taste buds was to steer you away from eating worthless or harmful things and direct you toward foods you need to stay healthy. You can't survive on calories alone. You need a variety of vital nutrients—vitamins, minerals, amino acids, and essential fatty acids. When you don't get enough of a particular nutrient, your body lets you know by causing you to crave foods that contain the missing substance. Food cravings are nature's way of preventing nutritional deficiencies.

Food cravings are the nemesis of all weight loss diets. A good example is the radical low-carbohydrate Atkins diet. The reason people couldn't stick with it was not hunger. Remember, you could eat all the calories you wanted. The problem was food cravings— yearning for the foods that were missing. Dieters missed the tartness and crispness of fruits and vegetables and the taste of sweets. After a few weeks, food cravings drove most Atkins dieters back to their old ways.

Low-fat diets cause even worse cravings. At least low-carb diets let you satisfy your hunger, but low-fat diets require you to consciously restrict calories in addition to reducing fat. In addition to craving your favorite fat-containing foods, you get just plain hungry. And if you succeed in reducing the fat in your diet, you tend to compensate by overeating other foods. That's usually not true of low-carbohydrate diets. When you reduce carbohydrates, you lower your insulin levels, which makes you naturally tend to eat less.

Most of the food humans eat contains some ingredient they need to stay healthy. Fresh fruit and vegetables contain vitamins, antioxidants, and fiber that are essential for good health. Humans who don't eat adequate amounts of fresh fruit and vegetables are susceptible to a host of nutritional problems, including scurvy, beriberi, and bowel problems. Animal products such as meat, dairy products, and eggs contain vitamins, iron, and protein, which you can't live without and are hard to get in other foods. People who don't get enough eggs, meat, or dairy products are subject to rickets, pernicious anemia, iron deficiency, and other diseases.

Although you can live without sugar, there's even a survival benefit of craving sweets. Most parts of plants are inedible, sometimes even poisonous, but parts that contain sugar, such as fruit or berries, are usually edible and nutritious. To prehistoric hunter-gatherers, sweetness was a sign that a plant part was safe to eat.

When you think of craving vital nutrients, you might think only of things that are absorbed into your bloodstream. However, humans also crave fiber, even though it passes through the digestive tract without getting absorbed. An agronomist once told me that he is occasionally summoned to a farm because the horses are eating wooden fence posts. If they don't get enough fiber in their feed, they start eating wood. Humans similarly crave crunchiness when they are deprived of fiber.

The point is that most of the foods we eat contain some ingredient that is vital for good health and creates natural cravings when taken away. Starch is the exception. It has no survival value other than to provide calories. It's virtually devoid of vitamins, minerals, antioxidants, amino acids, essential fatty acids, fiber, and anything else you need to stay healthy. There is no biological reason for craving it. No creature ever suffered any disease for lack of starch. Humans did fine for millions of years without it.

6

Sugar-Containing Beverages: Starch's Slippery Mimic

When it comes to releasing large amounts of sugar into your bloodstream, only one other common food—if you call it a food—comes close to starch, and that's sugar-sweetened beverages. Your digestive system breaks down starch to sugar and water, which is what sugar-sweetened beverages are to begin with. When you drink a sugary soft drink, you're doing the same thing you do when you eat starch: flooding your system with more glucose than it was designed to handle.

A teaspoon of sugar in your coffee or tea is not a problem. The glycemic load of a single teaspoon of sugar is only 28 percent of that of a slice of white bread. However, most sodas contain a lot more than a single teaspoon. A twelve-ounce can of Coca-Cola contains *ten* teaspoons of sugar.

Fortunately, most grown-ups who have diabetes or are concerned about their weight know enough to avoid nondiet sodas. But here's the bad news. Pop isn't the only culprit. Fruit juices, *even without added sugar,* are almost as bad. Think about it: if you take the sugar from several pieces of fruit and put it into one serving of juice, you have a sugar-sweetened beverage. A twelve-ounce serving of orange juice contains the equivalent of seven teaspoons of sugar. You might call the sugar in fruit juice "natural" because it comes from fruit, but it's sugar nonetheless. Your body doesn't know the difference between natural and added sugar. They both raise your blood sugar.

One of the reasons starch causes problems is that you can't taste the sugar in it. Only a small fraction of the sugar in starch is released in your mouth. Similarly, you can't taste most of the sugar in sugar-sweetened beverages, but for a different reason. Your mouth handles liquids differently from solids. You don't chew them. They pass over your tongue in a gulp without interacting with your taste buds. Indeed, we actually try to obscure the taste of sugar in beverages by adding sour ingredients such as lemon to offset the sugary taste, and by drinking them ice-cold, which further blunts the sweetness.

What's wrong with not tasting the sugar in beverages? As you recall from the previous chapter, sugar you taste satisfies your appetite more than sugar you don't taste. In one experiment, Purdue University researchers gave sugar in the form of jelly beans to a group of volunteers every day for four weeks and compared their daily food-eating patterns with that of a group given the same amount of calories in the form of a sugar-sweetened beverage. Those who ate the jelly beans usually reduced their food intake at their next meal, but those who consumed the sugar-containing beverage did not. At the end of four weeks, the subjects who had consumed the sugar in liquids gained weight, but those who had eaten sugar in solid candy did not. The bottom line is that sugar-sweetened beverages actually *add to,* rather than replace, calories from other foods. In a way, that's good news if you are a pop or juice drinker. It means you can eliminate a major source of calories from your diet without increasing your hunger for other foods.

Like the glucose in starch, the glucose in sugar-sweetened beverages enters your bloodstream much faster than glucose released by fresh fruit and vegetables. In fact, because your body has to break down starch to sugar and water before it can pass into your bloodstream, the sugar in liquids goes into your bloodstream even faster. Sugar-containing liquids raise blood sugar so consistently

Table 6.1   **Glycemic Loads of Common Beverages**

Beverage	Description	Glycemic Load (% of 1 slice of white bread)
Orange soda	12 oz. can	314
Gatorade	20 oz. bottle	273
Coca-Cola	12 oz. can	218
Cranberry juice	8 oz. glass	145
Pineapple juice, unsweetened	8 oz. glass	145
Raspberry smoothie	8 oz. glass	127
Orange juice	8 oz. glass	118
Apple juice, unsweetened	8 oz. glass	109
Grapefruit juice, unsweetened	8 oz. glass	100
Carrot juice	8 oz. glass	90
Chocolate milk	8 oz. glass	82
Soy milk	8 oz. glass	73
Tomato juice	8 oz. glass	36
Milk, skim	8 oz. glass	36
Milk, 2% fat	8 oz. glass	30

among people who are prone to diabetes that doctors often have patients drink a standardized mixture of sugar and water to test them for prediabetes.

Like starch, sugar-sweetened beverages are completely absorbed into the bloodstream in the first foot or two of intestine and never make it to the last part of the digestive tract, where several appetite-suppressing hormones are released. And like starch, sodas have no nutritive value other than providing calories. Because they contain no essential vitamins or minerals, eliminating them produces no biologically based craving. Fruit juices contain vitamins and minerals, but none that aren't plentiful in fresh fruit and vegetables.

As you can see in Table 6.1, when it comes to giving your system a glucose shock, sugar-sweetened beverages are right up there with bread, potatoes, and rice. Actually, sodas and fruit juices are even worse than their glycemic loads would indicate. Much of the sugar in them is *fructose*, a type of sugar that isn't measured by blood glucose tests.

Considering that sugar-sweetened beverages behave like starch once they enter your body, it's not surprising that they raise the risk of obesity and diabetes. In a study reported in the *Journal of the American Medical Association* in 2004, researchers tracked the eating habits of 51,603 women and found that those who consumed one or more sodas daily increased their risk of diabetes by 80 percent compared with women who seldom drank them. After eight years, women who consumed sodas daily gained an average of twenty pounds, compared with three pounds for women who drank them only occasionally. This was also true to a lesser extent in women who drank fruit juice daily. They had a 20 percent greater risk of diabetes compared with women who drank fruit juice only occasionally.

In the 1970s, when Americans started consuming more starch, they also started drinking more soda and fruit juice. The reasons were similar. Americans previously drank more milk than sodas, but as with eggs, meat, and other dairy products, milk's healthful image suffered when doctors started raising concerns about cholesterol. Also, as with starch, technological advances reduced production costs relative to the fresh-produce alternative milk. Because of increased availability of the cheap sweetener known as high-fructose corn syrup, soft-drink manufacturers increased the serving size of their drinks. Previously sodas came in seven-ounce bottles. Now they're regularly consumed in sixteen-ounce bottles and even gigantic thirty-two-ounce "Big Gulp" containers.

Before the 1970s, fruit juice was a rare treat. Oranges were expensive and available only seasonally. If you wanted orange juice, you had to wait until orange-harvesting season to get oranges. Then you had to squeeze them by hand—a big job. It took several pieces of fruit to make one glass of juice. With the advent of cheap frozen concentrates, orange juice has become a household staple and a major contributor to glycemic load.

Kids these days drink several times more pop than they did thirty years ago, which has contributed significantly to the obesity epidemic in children. Until recently, type 2 diabetes was rare in kids, but in recent years, the incidence has skyrocketed. Many researchers believe that increased consumption of sugar-sweetened beverages has played a major role.

The Diet-Soda Question

You may have heard mixed messages about diet soda, but if you're a diabetic and you like sodas, diet pop can be a blessing. Because it contains little or no sugar, it doesn't raise blood glucose levels at all.

Although diet sodas now account for half of all sodas consumed in the United States, they haven't prevented the current epidemics of obesity and diabetes. Some scientists have expressed concern that diet drinks might contribute to weight gain in other ways besides directly adding calories or raising insulin levels. They worry that by stimulating the same taste buds that sugar does, diet drinks might blunt their sensitivity. Those taste buds might then require more stimulation to satisfy the craving for sweetness, which could lead to increased consumption of sweets. Nevertheless, simply in terms of raising your blood sugar, diet sodas are fine.

Fruit Versus Fruit Juice

Many fruits and vegetables contain enough sugar to raise blood glucose levels, but the sugar in them is encapsulated by cell walls, dispersed in soluble fiber, and accompanied by mild acidity, all of which slow its release into your bloodstream. Although type 1 diabetics who are markedly deficient of insulin need to be careful of fruit, the glycemic loads of most fruits are acceptable for type 2 diabetics to enjoy in moderation.

There's a biological reason for craving fruit. Most fruits contain generous amounts of vitamins, minerals, antioxidants, and fiber, which are vital to good health. The tongue has taste buds that respond to the tanginess that fruit provides. Some scientists believe the purpose of these receptors is to ensure the right balance of minerals in the diet. Indeed, fruit is the best dietary source of the mineral potassium, which is especially beneficial to people with adult-onset diabetes or prediabetes. Here's why. High blood pressure is common among people with type 2 diabetes and prediabetes and, if poorly controlled, can be especially harmful for them. Low dietary potassium intake raises the risk of high blood pressure, and regular fruit consumption can actually lower blood pressure.

Fruit also contains soluble fiber, which helps slow glucose absorption not only in the fruit itself but also in other food consumed with fruit. In addition, the peels of fruit provide insoluble fiber, which contributes to good bowel function.

Although fruit can be good for you if you have type 2 diabetes, fruit *juice* is another matter. When you make fruit into fruit juice, you convert a healthful food to an unhealthful one. Changing fruit from solid to liquid reduces its hunger-satisfying effect, and the healthful fiber gets left behind. The high concentrations of sugar in fruit juices nullify whatever benefits you might derive from the vitamins and minerals they contain.

Coffee, Tea, or Milk?

In the 1960s people used to joke about how often flight attendants had to repeat the question "Coffee, tea, or milk?" On commercial airline flights, those were your beverage options. Except for alcoholic drinks, Americans drank little else. As sodas and fruit juices have become more common, Americans have gotten fatter and more diabetic.

Indeed, maybe we should have stuck with coffee, tea, and milk. The glycemic loads of coffee and tea are negligible. Scientists have carefully studied the effects of coffee and tea consumption on health, including any possible relationship to diabetes. These beverages do not predispose to diabetes or obesity. In fact, Finnish researchers have found that heavy coffee drinkers have *less* than average diabetes.

Because milk contains the sugar lactose—sometimes referred to as "milk sugar"—in the past, low-carb dieters were told to avoid it. However, when scientists began measuring the effects of various carbohydrates on blood sugar, they found that the glycemic load of milk is surprisingly low—27 for an eight-ounce glass. Indeed, milk might even be good for you if you are prone to diabetes. Harvard researchers studied the beverage habits of more than 37,000 women and found that daily milk drinkers had 20 percent less diabetes and 17 percent less obesity than women who were not milk drinkers. It is unclear whether milk has a protective effect or is just a sign of a healthy lifestyle. Indeed, milk drinkers tend to drink fewer sugar-sweetened beverages. Whatever the reason, if you have diabetes or prediabetes, milk is a better choice than soda or fruit juice.

Alcoholic Drinks

Scientists who have studied the relationship of alcohol consumption to health have found that people who drink alcohol are no more prone to develop diabetes than people who do not. Because most of the sugar in beer, wine, and liquor is fermented into alcohol, these drinks don't raise blood sugar. Generally, it's OK for diabetics and prediabetics to drink alcohol in moderation. Of course, sugar-containing mixers such as nondiet tonic water, ginger ale, and cola will raise your blood sugar just a soda does.

A word of caution: although alcohol doesn't raise blood sugar, it supplies plenty of calories, so it can contribute to weight gain. Like sugar-sweetened beverages, alcoholic beverages before meals add to rather than replace calories from other foods. In addition, by blunting the sensation of fullness, one or two drinks before a meal can cause you to overeat.

Rethinking Beverages in General

We are the only creatures on earth who drink anything but water. In fact, our prehistoric ancestors probably didn't even drink much water. They didn't have cups or glasses, they undoubtedly had to get down on their hands and knees and gulp water from streams or puddles. They couldn't have consumed liquids with every meal as we do now.

Freshwater was scarce in many of the areas in which prehistoric humans roamed. They probably went for days without drinking fluids, but they didn't need to be constantly drinking, because there was plenty of water in the food they ate. Meat is approximately 60 percent water, and vegetation is about 90 percent water.

No one seems to know how the rumor that you should drink eight glasses of water a day got started. A comprehensive review of the medical literature reported in the *American Journal of Physiology* in 2002 found no evidence that drinking more water than you are naturally inclined to drink does anything but make you urinate a lot. Unless you have been sweating profusely, you get most of the water you need in the food you eat.

Your body has powerful hormonal mechanisms for controlling the amount of water in your system. Your pituitary gland, an organ at the base of your brain, senses the concentration of water in your blood. When you become even slightly dehydrated, it secretes the hormone *vasopressin,* which makes you thirsty and tells your kidneys to conserve water. Your body will tell you in no uncertain terms if you need to drink. People don't become dehydrated without experiencing compelling thirst. In thirty-five years of practicing medicine, I've never seen anyone become dehydrated as a result of being too busy to drink.

Your body also has powerful mechanisms for preventing you from accumulating *too much* water. Indeed, excess water in your system can actually be dangerous. If you drink more water than your body needs to maintain the right concentration of water in your system, your pituitary gland tells your kidneys to let go of water. Within a few minutes, the excess is excreted into your urine. Drinking more water than your body tells you to drink doesn't somehow wash out your system, as many people believe. All that fluid exits your body directly.

Ironically, excessive fluids can actually make you susceptible to dehydration. If you're constantly drinking, your kidneys forget how to conserve water so that when you're deprived of it, you get dehydrated more quickly. In a rare psychiatric condition called pathological water drinking, constant excessive consumption of fluids causes the person's kidneys to lose the capacity to conserve water. When such patients are deprived of water even for a brief period, they continue to urinate excessively and become dangerously dehydrated.

The notion that drinking water will fill your stomach and keep you from eating more is a fallacy. The opposite is true. Experimental animals that are deprived of water invariably reduce their food intake. In the *American Journal of Physiology* in 2005, University of Pittsburgh researchers reported that vasopressin—the hormone the pituitary gland secretes when the body is deprived of fluid—also curbs appetite.

If you're trying to reduce after-meal surges in blood sugar, there's actually an argument to be made for avoiding beverages with meals. Fluids speed up the liquefaction of food in your stomach, and the more liquefied your stomach contents are, the faster they get digested, and the more they raise your blood sugar. Some diabetes experts now recommend that people with diabetes drink beverages *between* rather than with meals.

Along with the myth that you need to drink eight glasses of water a day came the notion that bottled water is more healthful than tap water—an idea for which there is no proof whatsoever. One thing for sure is that both notions have been a boon to companies that sell bottled water. It's interesting that the brand name of the popular bottled water Evian is the word *naive* spelled backward.

7

The Starch-Vulnerable Individual: How Insulin Resistance Works

We all eat more starch than our bodies were designed to handle, but most of us don't get diabetes. Why are only some of us susceptible? The answer has to do with something called *insulin resistance*.

Unlike children and young people with type 1 diabetes, who are severely deficient of insulin, if you have adult-onset diabetes you probably make plenty of insulin—maybe several times the normal amounts. Insulin is a powerful hormone. A fraction of the amount many adult diabetics make could kill a normal person. Why doesn't all that insulin lower your blood sugar? There's only one explanation: *your body is resistant to the blood-sugar-lowering effects of insulin*. Indeed, scientists have confirmed that the kind of diabetes most of us adults get is brought on by loss of sensitivity to insulin, a condition called insulin resistance.

Insulin resistance goes on for years before your blood sugar rises and doctors make the diagnosis of type 2 diabetes. At first, your beta cells compensate for your body's loss of sensitivity to insulin by just making more of it. However, years of excessive insulin production cause your beta cells to virtually wear out from overuse. When they can no longer compensate, your blood sugar rises.

The First Step: Weight Gain

For years, doctors noticed that, unlike young people with type 1 diabetes, most adult-onset diabetics were overweight. Now they know why. Not only does insulin resistance bring on diabetes; it promotes obesity.

The discovery of links between insulin resistance and unwanted weight gain changed many scientists' thinking not only about diabetes but also about obesity. In the past, most doctors thought that obesity was simply a matter of self-indulgence—that overweight folks just can't resist eating more than their bodies tell them they need. Of course, nobody wants to be fat, so you had to assume that overweight individuals either lack willpower or had psychological problems. However, when psychologists got around to studying the matter, they found no psychological differences between overweight and normal-weight people. Indeed, many overweight people show remarkable self-discipline in other aspects of their lives.

Most scientists now believe that obesity is not a manifestation of weak willpower or psychological problems. Rather, it's caused by a hormonal disturbance that creates an imbalance between the amount of calories people need to quell a natural hunger and the amount they burn off. Considering that the incidence of obesity is much higher than it was thirty years ago, it is apparent that something about the modern lifestyle is triggering that hormonal disturbance in more people than ever.

The strongest known calorie-storing hormone is insulin. Doctors have known for years that excessive amounts of insulin given as medication cause weight gain. Researchers have recently discovered that most people who are thirty pounds overweight or more have insulin resistance, even if they don't have diabetes, and many scientists now believe that the large amounts of insulin produced by the body to compensate for insulin resistance promote obesity.

When you develop insulin resistance, not all parts of your body lose responsiveness to it equally. Some tissues shut down to insulin almost completely, while other tissues, particularly your fat cells, continue responding to it. Insulin is a powerful calorie-storing hormone. It pushes calories into fat deposits, and many scientists believe that's the problem. As discussed in the previous chapter, excessive amounts of insulin act to lock calories into your fat cells so your body can't use them for energy—a phenomenon scientists call "internal starvation." This causes the frustrating paradox of obesity: even though you have several weeks' worth of calories stored up in your body fat, you're as hungry as ever.

Your body needs only small amounts of insulin to handle non-starchy foods such as meat, dairy products, and fresh fruit and vegetables. Almost all of the insulin modern humans produce is in response to eating starch—grain products, potatoes, rice, and corn. Indeed, the Nurses' Health Study found that the glycemic load of the starches in the average American's diet is several times higher than that of all of the other foods combined. By causing people's bodies to produce excessive insulin, amounts of starch typical of the modern diet cause many of us to gain unwanted weight.

Most people who do not have insulin resistance can consume amounts of starch typical of the modern diet without getting fat or developing diabetes; but for individuals who have insulin resistance, starch is a toxin. By causing the body to overproduce insulin, it leads to excess fat accumulation and, in some folks, to beta-cell exhaustion and diabetes.

Although people with insulin resistance frequently develop weight problems when they consume amounts of starch typical of the modern diet, only some of them get diabetes. Their beta cells continue making enough insulin to compensate for the body's loss of sensitivity to it. Why some people's beta cells wear out sooner than those of others is unclear, although genetics plays a role.

Insulin Resistance: a Muscle Problem

Insulin resistance is not exactly a disease. It's better described as a common variation in the ability of people's bodies to handle carbohydrates. According to researchers, about 22 percent of the American population has insulin resistance; among Americans older than fifty, that figure rises to 40 percent.

Insulin resistance tends to run in families. Yale University scientists discovered differences in the way family members of type 2 diabetics metabolize carbohydrates years before they gain weight or develop diabetes.

The genetic tendency toward insulin resistance is more common in some ethnic groups than in others. For example, the incidence is higher among people of Asian and African descent than among those of European heritage. Insulin resistance is especially common among Native Americans and Pacific Islanders. In general, the less time in its history an ethnic group has had to adapt to a starch-based diet, the higher the incidence of insulin resistance.

Your muscles are by far your body's biggest users of sugar. Insulin resistance is mainly a problem of loss of sensitivity of your muscles to insulin. Although heredity sets the stage for insulin resistance, the chief cause is lack of physical activity. Regardless of genetics, people who are physically active usually do not become insulin resistant. Indeed, among family members of type 2 diabetics, those who exercise regularly develop diabetes less than half as often as those who don't.

What's remarkable about the relationship of exercise to insulin resistance is how little physical activity it takes to restore insulin sensitivity. Walking just twenty minutes every other day has a significant protective effect against type 2 diabetes and obesity. The problem is that these days many of us don't even do that much exercise. Mechanization has taken over much of the physical activities people previously had to do to survive. The relationship between exercise and insulin sensitivity will be discussed further in Chapter 12.

The Obesity–Insulin Resistance Cycle

There's one more common contributor to insulin resistance: obesity itself. It's a vicious cycle: insulin resistance promotes weight gain, which causes more insulin resistance. This explains why it's so easy to gain weight and so hard to lose it. The good news is that the cycle also runs in reverse. Insulin is the key. If you eliminate starch, your body produces less insulin, which promotes weight loss, which improves insulin sensitivity, so your body produces even less insulin. This is why low-carbohydrate diets are so effective for losing weight.

"Metabolic Syndrome," or "Syndrome X"

Measuring insulin sensitivity directly is a complicated procedure that can be done only in specialized research laboratories. However, doctors have learned that they can diagnose insulin resistance by looking for the following signs:

- A tendency to accumulate fat in the abdomen
- High blood levels of triglyceride
- Low blood levels of good cholesterol (HDL)
- Borderline or high blood pressure
- Borderline blood sugar readings

For years before doctors knew about insulin resistance, they noticed that people who had one of the signs just listed usually had one or two of the others, and that such individuals were prone to heart attacks. They called the clustering of more than one of those characteristics in a single individual the "metabolic syndrome" or "syndrome X." Scientists now know that what causes these signs to occur together is insulin resistance. If you have two or more of those signs, more likely than not you have insulin resistance. A better name would be the "insulin resistance syndrome," but the term *metabolic syndrome* seems to have stuck.

Gauging How Insulin Resistant You Are

While it is difficult to measure insulin sensitivity directly, the more of those findings you have and the more pronounced they are, the worse your insulin resistance is likely to be. Here's how to use those signs to gauge how insulin resistant you are:

A tendency to gain weight in the abdomen. People who are insulin resistant often have what's commonly called a potbelly. Scientists aren't sure if insulin resistance causes fat to accumulate in the abdomen in preference to other parts of the body or if fat in the abdomen causes insulin resistance. Either way, the best indicator of how insulin resistant you are is your abdominal girth. (This is different from your pants size. To determine your abdominal girth, measure the circumference of your abdomen at the level of your navel with a tape measure.) An abdominal girth of thirty-eight inches for men or thirty-four inches for women doubles the risk of type 2 diabetes. A girth of forty inches for men or thirty-six inches for women triples the risk. A girth of forty-two inches for men or thirty-eight inches for women quadruples the risk.

Some people with insulin resistance actually look slim. They might not have much fat on their hips, arms, and legs. Sometimes the only sign is a belly that is disproportionate to the size of their buttocks. An abdominal girth greater than 95 percent of hip circumference in men or 85 percent in women suggests insulin resistance, even if body weight is normal.

High blood triglyceride level. When your body is having trouble dealing with the carbohydrates in your diet, your liver converts the excess glucose to fat, packages up the fat in particles called *triglycerides*, and sends them through your bloodstream to your fat deposits. The level of triglyceride in your blood is a good indicator of how insulin resistant you are. (Doctors routinely measure triglycerides when they check cholesterol. You can probably find out what your blood triglyceride level is by calling your doctor's office.) A fasting blood triglyceride level of 150 or more or an after-meal reading of 175 or more suggests insulin resistance. Most doctors regard fasting triglyceride levels of 150 to 200 as mild elevations, levels of 200 to 250 as moderate rises, and levels greater than 250 as marked increases.

Triglyceride levels fluctuate from day to day. Because a day or two of avoiding starch and exercising will usually lower your blood triglyceride significantly, your fasting levels might be normal even if you have insulin resistance. Triglyceride levels are actually more sensitive at detecting insulin resistance if they are measured about four hours after eating a starch-containing meal.

Low blood levels of "good cholesterol." HDL, otherwise known as "good cholesterol," protects your arteries from cholesterol buildup. However, high levels of triglycerides in your blood deplete good cholesterol. In addition to being a risk factor for cholesterol buildup in arteries, low HDL levels are a sign of insulin resistance. Because HDL levels take a few weeks to change, a low HDL level suggests that your triglyceride level has been high even though you might have measured the triglyceride level when it was temporarily normal. An HDL level less than 40 for men or less than 50 for women suggests insulin resistance.

Because genes strongly influence good cholesterol levels, you might have a normal HDL reading despite insulin resistance. On the other hand, it might be low in the absence of insulin resistance. In addition, exercise and alcohol raise HDL levels, and cigarette smoking lowers them.

Borderline or high blood pressure. Insulin resistance raises blood pressure slightly. These elevations are often so mild they pass as insignificant. Normally your blood pressure should be 120/80 or less. Although most doctors don't pay much attention to readings lower than 140/90, insulin-resistant individuals usually have levels that are slightly higher than 120/80. Blood pressure readings of 130/85 or more strongly correlate with insulin resistance even if they don't exceed 140/90, a level most doctors would call high.

Borderline blood sugar readings. If you have type 2 diabetes, you already know that your blood sugar is higher than normal. However, if you're like most people with type 2 diabetes, you probably had borderline readings for years before you were finally diagnosed with diabetes. In the absence of diabetes, a fasting blood sugar reading greater than 110 or a level greater than 140 after a meal suggests insulin resistance.

Although most people with adult-onset diabetes have a combination of insulin resistance and beta-cell failure, the relative contributions of each vary. Some adult-onset diabetics make a lot of insulin but are very resistant to its effects. Others are more sensitive to insulin, but their beta cells make less of it. It's useful to gauge the amount of insulin resistance you have because treatment to relieve insulin resistance differs in some ways from treatment to correct insulin deficiency. The relative contributions of these two disturbances will determine which medicines and lifestyle changes will work best to control your diabetes.

As discussed earlier, you can estimate how insulin resistant you are by considering how many of the signs of metabolic syndrome you have and how severe they are. Once you have an idea of how insulin resistant you are, you can gauge how well your beta cells are working by considering how high your blood sugar is in relationship to your insulin resistance. For example, if you have signs of severe insulin resistance but your blood sugar is only mildly elevated, your beta cells probably function pretty well. On the other hand, if you have only subtle signs of insulin resistance but very high blood sugar readings, your beta cells have probably lost much of their capacity to make insulin.

Here are some real-life examples of patients of mine with type 2 diabetes who needed different approaches to treatment because of differences in the relative contributions of insulin resistance and beta cell failure.

Judy

At the age of thirty-seven, during a routine examination by her gynecologist, Judy learned she had high blood sugar. She had gained sixty-five pounds since high school. She was frustrated by her weight but otherwise felt fine. On examination, she showed flagrant signs of insulin resistance. She had a typical "potbelly" physique. Her abdominal girth was thirty-nine inches. Her arms, legs, and buttocks were comparatively slim. Her fasting blood sugar was only mildly increased at 154, but her triglyceride level was quite high at 240, her HDL level was low at 38, and her blood pressure was elevated at 138/86.

Considering that Judy's blood sugar was only mildly increased despite signs of severe insulin resistance, she was probably mak-

ing plenty of insulin. Her main problem was loss of sensitivity to insulin. Medication to increase her insulin levels might have lowered her blood sugar but would have worsened her tendency to gain weight. Emphasis needed to be placed on reducing her needs for insulin by improving her body's sensitivity to insulin with insulin-sensitizing medications and exercise.

Tom

Tom's doctor discovered diabetes during a routine examination at age fifty-one. He had gained twenty pounds since high school. He was physically active at his job and managed to play a couple of rounds of golf a week. Although he had a slight potbelly, he was only mildly overweight. His abdominal girth was thirty-seven inches. His fasting blood sugar was 260, triglyceride 170, and blood pressure 126/84.

Tom showed only subtle signs of insulin resistance. His physically active lifestyle helped prevent it. However, his fasting blood sugar was markedly elevated. Lack of insulin probably played a larger role in Tom's case than in Judy's. Relatively more emphasis needed to be placed on ensuring adequate levels of insulin than on increasing insulin sensitivity.

Whereas Tom and Judy required somewhat different approaches to treatment, both benefited from eliminating starch. In Judy's case, in addition to lowering her blood sugar, it helped reduce the amount of insulin she needed, which helped her lose weight and further sensitize her body to insulin. In Tom's case, cutting out starch brought his carbohydrate intake in line with his beta cells' reduced capacity to make insulin.

"Type 1.5 Diabetes"

Most adult-onset diabetics have insulin resistance. Indeed, loss of sensitivity to insulin combined with excessive dietary starch is what brings on type 2 diabetes. However, some people with adult-onset diabetes show no signs of insulin resistance. They aren't overweight, and their triglyceride, HDL, and blood pressure levels are normal. Many of these individuals actually have an adult form of type 1 diabetes. Their beta cells have been damaged by an immune reaction, as in childhood diabetes, rather than overwork, as they are in type 2 diabetes. Doctors call this "type 1.5 diabetes" or latent autoimmune diabetes in adults (LADA). These patients don't benefit much from treatment to relieve insulin resistance. They mainly need to replace the missing insulin with insulin medication.

Type 2 Diabetes in Kids

It usually takes years of insulin resistance and heavy starch consumption to wear out a person's beta cells, which is why type 2 diabetes usually doesn't come on until middle age. Until lately, this kind of diabetes was rare in young people. However, in recent years, along with increasing numbers of obese children, doctors are seeing more young people with the adult-onset kind of diabetes. Like middle-aged diabetics, these overweight kids have severe insulin resistance and are already starting to wear out their beta cells. Sugar-sweetened beverages and confections play a larger role in causing diabetes in kids than they do in adults.

8

Things That Get Better When You Eliminate Starch

Until recently, starches—grains, potatoes, rice, and corn—were considered indispensable parts of the American diet. But once scientists began questioning the notion that starches are harmless "empty calories" and started looking for links between refined carbohydrates and diseases, they discovered connections between starch consumption and several previously puzzling medical conditions, including obesity, diabetes, heart and blood vessel disease, female infertility, acne, age-related vision loss, and even some cancers. The good news is that eliminating starch can prevent, improve, or cure those conditions in addition to alleviating several bothersome symptoms that affect most people. Here's what happens when you remove starch from your diet:

• **You often lose weight without dieting.** As discussed in Chapter 5, insulin is a potent calorie-storing hormone. It pushes calories into your fat depots. Excessive amounts of insulin, whether produced by your body or taken as medication, prevent calories from being released from your fat cells. Even though you have plenty of calories stored up as fat, you seem to be hungry all of the time. When you eliminate starch, insulin levels fall, and your body starts tapping into your fat depots for energy. You eat less because you have access to your own calorie stores, which allows you to lose weight without consciously cutting calories.

What's remarkable about eliminating starch is not just that you lose more weight than you do with other kinds of diets, but that *you lose it without trying to reduce the amount of food you eat.* Study after study has shown that people who eliminate carbohydrates without trying to cut calories lose more weight than those on low-fat diets who *try* to cut calories.

Cutting out starch works especially well for people with high blood levels of insulin either produced naturally or taken as medication. That includes most adult-onset diabetics, prediabetics, and overweight persons. Of the dozens of weight-loss programs reported in the medical literature, by far the best results have been among type 2 diabetics who eliminated starch. As reported in the journal *Nutrition and Metabolism,* Swedish researchers instructed a group of patients with adult-onset diabetes who were overweight to follow a low-starch diet and compared them with a similar group of diabetics who continued to consume typical amounts of carbohydrates. The group who followed the low-starch diet lost an average of 25 pounds. Unlike many diets reported in the medical literature, in which much of the weight was regained within a year, these patients had kept their weight off two years later when the study ended. No other weight loss diet study in the recent medical literature has reported results that good.

• **If you don't already have diabetes, you will reduce your risk of getting it.** Excessive demands for insulin ultimately can wear out your insulin-making cells. Cutting out starch relieves the burden on those cells and forestalls diabetes. Harvard researchers analyzed the diets of 85,059 nurses and checked on their health twenty years later. The nurses who consumed a low-starch diet developed diabetes less than half as often as those whose diet was high in starch. Although the women who consumed less starch gained less weight, obesity prevention wasn't the only factor. The diabetes rate was lower in women who consumed less starch even among those who gained weight. Lowering the body's demands for insulin, regardless of weight loss, reduced the burden on these women's insulin-producing cells and prevented those cells from wearing out.

- **If you have diabetes, it will improve dramatically.** Your body doesn't need much insulin to handle low-glycemic-load foods like eggs, meat, dairy products, nuts, and fresh fruit and vegetables. Most of the insulin the average American makes is in response to eating starch. If you cut out flour products, potatoes, rice, soft drinks, and juices, even if you don't reduce the number of calories you take in, you reduce the glycemic load of your diet to a fraction of what it was. If you have diabetes, this will have a profound effect on your blood sugar and your body's requirements for insulin. A warning: *if you take insulin, you should not attempt to reduce the starch content of your diet without first reducing your insulin dose.* In the Swedish study just described, among the patients who followed a low-starch diet, the average insulin dose needed to control their diabetes fell from 60 to 18 units per day. Some of those patients were able to stop taking insulin altogether.

- **You will eliminate after-meal spikes in your blood sugar.** Even if your fasting blood sugar readings are normal, after-meal surges in your blood sugar can harm your blood vessels. Many diabetes experts believe that exaggerated blood sugar fluctuations are as harmful as sustained high blood sugar.

Although doctors have lots of good medication for lowering fasting blood sugar levels, it's more difficult to control after-meal surges. Doctors sometimes instruct patients to give themselves shots of rapid-acting insulin at meals to control these spikes. Although this approach can help, it's fraught with problems. It's difficult to predict exactly what a starchy meal will do to your blood sugar or the timing with which it will do it. How high your blood sugar goes depends on a host of factors, including not only the glycemic load of the carbohydrates you eat but also the kinds of foods you eat with them, the order in which you eat them, and your activities before and afterward. Consequently, it's easy to misjudge the amount of insulin you need. If the dose is too low, your blood sugar will shoot up too high. If the dose is too high, the blood sugar could fall to dangerously low levels.

There's only one sure way to avoid after-meal blood sugar surges: *don't eat foods that raise blood sugar in the first place.* If you stick to low-glycemic-load foods, you can eat freely without your blood sugar rising too much afterward.

- **The cholesterol in your blood will become less harmful.** High levels of cholesterol in your blood can build up in the walls of your arteries and cause damage. However, you can have normal cholesterol levels and still end up with cholesterol buildup. In fact, most heart attack victims do not have particularly high cholesterol levels.

Whether the cholesterol in your blood causes damage to your arteries depends more on the balance between your good and bad cholesterol levels than on your bad cholesterol alone. If you have insulin resistance, excessive dietary starch increases blood triglyceride levels and reduces levels of good cholesterol, which makes the bad cholesterol in your blood more damaging.

Genes more than diet determine the level of bad cholesterol in your blood. Contrary to popular belief, neither low-cholesterol diets nor exercise lowers blood levels of bad cholesterol much. However, if you cut out starch, especially if you also engage in moderate exercise, you can sharply reduce your triglyceride levels and raise *good*-cholesterol levels, which prevents bad cholesterol from damaging your arteries.

- **You will reduce your risk of heart disease.** Buildup of cholesterol in the arteries that supply blood to the heart, the *coronary arteries*, is the leading cause of death of Americans and Europeans. The four main risk factors for coronary artery disease are imbalances between good and bad cholesterol, high blood pressure, cigarette smoking, and high blood glucose levels. Excessive dietary starch increases blood glucose levels, worsens imbalances between good and bad cholesterol, and raises blood pressure. In other words, it worsens three of the four major risk factors for heart disease.

Lowering glycemic load prevents heart attacks. Researchers at the University of Montreal gave 714 type 2 diabetics acarbose—a drug that slows the absorption of starch, thereby decreasing its glycemic load—and compared their heart attack rate with that of 715 similar patients who did not get the drug. The group that took acarbose ended up with lower blood pressure levels, lower triglyceride levels, higher levels of good cholesterol, and an astounding 90 percent lower rate of heart attacks.

- **If you have polycystic ovary syndrome, it will improve.** One of the most common, distressing, and underdiagnosed medical conditions that affect women is a menstrual disorder called polycystic ovary syndrome (PCOS). It causes cysts in the ovaries, irregular periods, infertility, acne, unwanted body hair, and obesity. Approximately 28 percent of women who are overweight have PCOS.

Until recently, the cause of PCOS eluded physicians. In the 1990s, some PCOS patients who happened to be taking the insulin-sensitizing medication metformin noticed that their PCOS symptoms improved soon after starting the drug. Their periods became regular, and some of them became pregnant. Scientists soon discovered that the same thing that brings on type 2 diabetes—overproduction of insulin—also brings on polycystic ovary syndrome. Later studies showed that virtually all women who have PCOS have severe insulin resistance. In addition to weight gain, excessive insulin production causes these women to develop ovarian cysts, menstrual difficulties, and infertility.

In the past, PCOS was considered primarily a fertility problem and was handled mainly by gynecologists. Other doctors knew little about it. Gynecologists generally don't treat many patients with type 2 diabetes, so they were late in learning about insulin resistance. Consequently, PCOS has been one of the most misunderstood, underdiagnosed, and undertreated conditions that affect women. Many doctors still fail to recognize PCOS when dealing with related problems of obesity and menstrual irregularities.

When women consult doctors about unwanted weight gain, often the only condition the women get tested for is an underactive thyroid gland, which rarely turns out to be the problem.

PCOS is not just a problem for women of childbearing age. The tendency for starch to cause excessive insulin secretion and weight gain in these women continues for life and makes them especially vulnerable to type 2 diabetes. Approximately 25 percent of women with PCOS eventually develop diabetes.

Polycystic ovary syndrome can be treated by reducing the body's demands for insulin with insulin-sensitizing drugs, exercise, and avoidance of starch.

• **You may reduce the risk of age-related vision loss.** Recently, scientists discovered a link between dietary starch and *age-related macular degeneration* (AMD), now the most common cause of vision loss in old age. Because this finding is new and macular degeneration takes years to develop, no studies have been done yet to determine if reducing starch consumption can prevent or reverse AMD.

• **Your skin will clear up.** Acne, or "pimples," is caused by inflammation of the skin's oil glands. Doctors have long suspected a relationship between diet and acne, but have never been able to pin it down. Recently, scientists discovered that diets high in starch change the composition of the oil these glands produce in a way that makes those oils more susceptible to bacterial degradation. When researchers instructed acne patients to follow a low-glycemic-load diet, they developed significantly fewer pimples compared with those who continued eating typical amounts of starch.

• **You will prevent *low* blood sugar.** It may seem strange that something that causes high blood sugar also causes *low* blood sugar, or *hypoglycemia,* but when you eat something starchy, your blood sugar will often rise abruptly, then reverse course and fall too low, a condition called *reactive hypoglycemia.*

When large amounts of glucose enter your bloodstream all at once, your body can't fine-tune its insulin response as well as it can to glucose that trickles in slowly. Insulin secretion often overshoots and drives the blood sugar down too far. Low blood sugar causes a feeling of weakness, poor concentration, jitteriness, and hunger, all of which are promptly relieved by eating something starchy or sugary.

Reactive hypoglycemia is especially likely to affect you if you have prediabetes or insulin resistance, because your beta cells have to produce more insulin than normal in response to eating starch. Indeed, reactive hypoglycemia is one of the first signs of insulin resistance.

It is the body's response to rapidly falling blood sugar, rather than low blood sugar itself, that causes most of the symptoms of low blood sugar. Your body has several mechanisms for preventing low blood sugar. When it senses that your blood sugar level is falling too fast, it releases hormones that quickly raise it back up. One of these hormones, *adrenaline*, causes much of the tremulousness, apprehension, and inability to concentrate that accompany hypoglycemia.

Considering that the normal human body sometimes has trouble producing the right amount of insulin to handle starch, it's not surprising that diabetics trying to figure out how much insulin to take have even more trouble. Insulin is a powerful hormone. It will always lower your blood sugar if you take enough of it. The problem is that if you take too much insulin, your blood sugar will fall too far. Unlike reactive hypoglycemia, which is usually mild and harmless, hypoglycemia caused by taking too much insulin medication can cause confusion, coma, and even death. Indeed, the possibility of low blood sugar from taking too much insulin is the biggest challenge to maintaining good blood sugar control with insulin.

Here's where something called the "law of small numbers" comes in. If you keep your glycemic load small, your blood sugar spikes will be small, and the amount of insulin you need to control your blood sugar will be small. Then if you misjudge a little, your body's natural defenses against hypoglycemia can compensate. Eliminating starch makes it easier to take insulin because it reduces the danger of hypoglycemia.

• **You will feel better.** Most people don't feel anything when their blood sugar rises. It's two or three hours afterward, when it falls too fast, that you experience tremulousness, weakness, irritability, and compelling hunger. Eating a starchy snack will quickly relieve those symptoms but start the cycle over again. Highs and lows of blood sugar throughout the day can leave you feeling edgy and exhausted. People with insulin resistance are especially prone to these symptoms.

Long before scientists discovered insulin resistance, doctors knew that eating more protein and less starch for breakfast prevents midmorning reactive hypoglycemia. However, sometime in the 1950s or '60s, Americans went from having eggs and meat for breakfast to eating starchy stuff like breakfast cereals, toast, and bagels. Starting the day with a glucose shock sets the cycles of high and low blood sugar in motion. Several studies have shown that starchy breakfasts cause people to consume more calories throughout the day than do starch-free ones.

• **Your mental performance will improve.** In addition to causing irritability and fatigue, fluctuating blood sugar levels affect mental performance. Scientists at the University of Edinburgh gave subjects insulin shots to lower their blood sugar, and then measured what psychologists call *working memory*, the mental processes you use to hold a sequence of steps in your memory long enough to carry them out. For example, if you think of a series of thngs you want to enter into your computer, your working memory allows you to hold them in mind long enough to type them in. The scientists found that low blood sugar of the degree that often occurs following a starchy meal can markedly impair (they used the word *obliterate*) working memory.

If your working memory isn't up to par, you might find yourself stopping in the middle of mental tasks to recall what you were trying to do. If your job requires performing such routines repetitively throughout the day, poor working memory takes a toll on your efficiency. People in occupations that require sustained mental focus, such as computer programmers, often report periods of poor concentration that occur when they haven't eaten for a few hours. Their performance improves when they eat, but if the snack is starchy, which it often tends to be, it sets them up for another round of reactive hypoglycemia. The worker eventually learns to have a snack to head off the symptoms. Snacking throughout the day combined with the sedentary nature of such work makes people in those occupations particularly susceptible to weight gain and diabetes.

- **Your physical performance will improve.** Starch also affects physical performance. People engaged in endurance sports such as long-distance running or cycling sometimes complain of "hitting the wall," a wave of fatigue that occurs after forty-five minutes or so of continuous exertion. This sensation, also known as "bonking," often correlates with a slight drop in blood sugar—not enough to cause hypoglycemia but apparently, for some people, enough to make exercise seem harder.

Many athletes say that a carbohydrate snack during exercise relieves bonking. Cyclists often use a banana or an energy drink for that purpose. This has spawned the notion that "carb loading," eating starchy food before exercise, will prevent bonking. Although there is actually some truth to this, it's tricky. Eating carbohydrates the night before an athletic event will help ensure that your glucose stores are filled to capacity, which, in theory, could be beneficial. However, loading up on starch or sugar just before exercise can produce an outpouring of insulin that makes the blood sugar fall more during exercise.

Here's why reducing dietary starch can relieve bonking. Muscles are able to use both fat and glucose to do their work. However, if you constantly flood your body with glucose from the food you eat, your muscles become less efficient at burning fat for fuel and adapted to burning more glucose instead. As a result, when you exercise, your muscles use up glucose faster, which depletes your limited glucose stores sooner and makes your blood sugar fall more. If you reduce the starch in your diet for a couple of weeks, your muscles become better able to use fat instead of glucose for energy, which lessens the drop in blood sugar that occurs after prolonged exercise.

- **And remember, there is no downside to eliminating starch.** Starch provides no known benefit to humans other than supplying calories. In amounts typical of the diets of modern humans, starch causes or aggravates several serious and frustrating medical conditions, and reducing dietary starch prevents, improves, or cures those conditions. If you're overweight or have diabetes or prediabetes, cutting it out of your diet can do nothing but help you.

9

Kicking the Addiction

You're addicted when you know something you're doing is causing you trouble but you keep doing it anyway. By that definition, a lot of us are addicted to starch and probably a few other things. But substances that are truly addictive—alcohol or heroin, for example—produce physical dependence. If you use them regularly, you experience uncomfortable symptoms when you try to stop. Taking more of the drug relieves those symptoms, so you get into a cycle of gratification followed by "withdrawal" symptoms that trigger craving for more of the drug.

Most addictive drugs work by overstimulating normal physiological pathways. Heroin, for example, stimulates nervous-system pathways responsible for relieving pain, which produces intense pleasure. The problem is that overloading those circuits causes them to malfunction when the drug wears off, which produces unpleasant symptoms, such as anxiety, shakiness, and sweating.

By no means is starch as physically addictive as alcohol or heroin, but it produces a similar addictive cycle. By overloading pathways that metabolize carbohydrates, starch causes your body to produce large amounts of insulin. Excessive insulin locks calories into your fat stores so that a couple hours after eating, you're hungry again. Sometimes the insulin surge is so strong that it triggers low blood sugar, which causes nervousness and jitteriness not unlike withdrawal from an addictive drug. Like an addict needing a fix, you're craving more of the substance that started the cycle in the first place. In one experiment, scientists gave subjects insulin to lower their blood sugar and then observed the kinds of foods they chose to eat. Sure enough, low blood sugar gave them a preference for starch.

Starch's Long-Term Addictive Effects

As unpleasant as withdrawing from heroin or alcohol can be, most of the distressing physical effects of withdrawal—anxiety, shakiness, sweating—dissipate in a week or two. The need to take drugs to relieve uncomfortable physical symptoms subsides. However, the tendency toward addiction doesn't go away. Chronic alcohol and drug use has long-lasting effects on the mind and body that increase the likelihood of returning to the addictive cycle. Typically, one dose of the drug can set it off.

Similarly, years of excessive starch consumption sensitize people's bodies to starch's addictive effects. As long as they avoid refined carbohydrates, their urge to eat starch diminishes, but if they start eating it again, they often don't stop. Like alcoholics who fall off the wagon, they fall back into the addictive cycle.

The culprit is insulin resistance. Reduced sensitivity to insulin causes the body to produce more than normal amounts of insulin to handle even small amounts of starch, which makes people vulnerable to starch's addictive effects long after they have reduced their intake of it.

Compared with the cycles of euphoria and withdrawal that drugs such as alcohol or heroin produce, starch's addictive cycle is easy to break. A few days of avoiding starch and eating more fat, protein, and fresh fruits and vegetables stabilizes blood sugar and reduces insulin levels. In addition, exercise improves the body's sensitivity to insulin, so you don't have to make so much insulin to handle carbohydrates. As little as two or three days of avoiding starch and just walking a half hour a day allows calories to be mobilized from fat depots, staves off between-meal hunger, and reduces starch cravings.

Starch as Comfort Food

There's more to drug and alcohol addiction than relieving withdrawal symptoms. People use these substances to improve their mood—in effect, to alter their perception of reality. The mood-altering effects of eating starch are minor compared with those produced by alcohol or drugs and obviously don't affect behavior or judgment the way those chemicals do. Nevertheless, eating has a calming, mood-lifting effect, which people often use to relax or relieve stress. Indeed, scientists have found that eating temporarily reduces blood levels of stress hormones associated with anxiety and depression.

People who snack for relaxation or to relieve stress often prefer specific foods commonly called "comfort foods" for that purpose. Although these are often refined carbohydrates, carbs are not necessarily most people's favorites. Psychologists have found that the important quality for a comfort food is that it has pleasant associations. Some people claim soups, casseroles, and even meat as their favorite comfort food. People turn to refined carbohydrates mainly because they're convenient.

The secret to preventing the comfort food habit from raising your blood sugar is to do a little advance planning. Comfort food eating is usually impulsive; little thought goes into it. You can keep it from raising your blood sugar by just making sure something besides refined carbohydrates—for example, nuts, fruit, or cheese—is available when the urge strikes.

How to Satisfy a Starch Tooth Without Eating Starch

Let's face it. It's not just physical addiction or the need for comfort food that makes people eat starch. Folks like the taste. But if starch is largely tasteless, what's there to like?

Although starch is 98 percent flavorless, it isn't completely so. Enzymes in saliva break down about 2 percent of it to sugar, which you can taste. Thus, a "starch tooth" is largely a sweet tooth. Indeed, humans are hardwired to respond to sugar. Humans have taste buds specifically devoted to detecting sweetness. When hunter-gatherers tasted a plant to see if it was edible, sweetness indicated that it was a safe source of calories.

Because a starch tooth is actually a sweet tooth, you can satisfy the urge for starch by eating something sweet but not starchy—for example, a piece of chocolate. But wait! Aren't sweets forbidden if you have diabetes? Indeed, if you ate a portion of chocolate as large as a typical portion of bread, potatoes, or rice, it would release about the same amount of sugar into your bloodstream. The difference is that most people don't eat as much chocolate at one time as they do bread, potatoes, or rice. You don't need much chocolate just to satisfy your urge for something sweet.

Sugar can actually be your friend if you have diabetes. It's easier to pass up the bread, potatoes, and rice at dinner if you can look forward to something sweet for dessert. The trick is to use sugar to satisfy the urge for sweetness, *not* to satisfy hunger. After a meal, you should be full. You should use candy only to satisfy your urge for something sweet. If you're really still hungry, you should have some more meat or vegetables. A good rule of thumb is to limit the amount of sweets you eat for dessert to no more than you can wrap the fingers of one hand around. You should consume sweets only after a meal, not by themselves. Pure chocolate, chocolate-covered nuts, a few jelly beans, or a piece of hard candy would be OK. Cookies and cakes are out because they're mainly starch.

A word of caution: although most adults don't overeat candy, there are notable exceptions. Some people respond to sugar as if it were an addictive drug. Stimulation of their sweetness receptors seems to set off an addictive cycle of its own. These individuals might finish a box of chocolates in one sitting. If you're one of those people, you're better off abstaining from sweets altogether.

Although starch consumption has risen dramatically in the past thirty years, along with the diabetes and obesity rate, Americans have not increased their consumption of candy. Indeed, when investigators tried to study the effects of a high-sugar diet, they found that it was difficult to get subjects to eat more sugar than they were naturally inclined to. That's certainly not true of starch. Scientists have no trouble getting folks to eat double or triple their usual daily portions of starch.

While we naturally crave a little stimulation of our sweetness receptors, some of us prefer the subtle sweetness of starch to the more intense stimulation of candy. If you just want gentle stimulation of your sweetness receptors, other sweet foods besides starch can do the job without worsening your diabetes. Fresh fruit is usually OK. Although some fruits raise blood sugar a little, their effects are minor compared with those of refined carbohydrates. Nuts are especially good substitutes for starch. They impart a subtle sweetness and have a dry, crunchy texture reminiscent of a starchy snack. Their high protein and "good fat" content satisfies hunger with negligible effects on blood sugar or insulin levels. Indeed, nuts have been part of the human diet for millions of years.

Confronting the Economic Addiction

It would be difficult to sober up if the only liquids in the world were beer, wine, and gin. That's what it might seem like when you try to cut out starch. Even if you're not interested in eating it, it's foisted upon you at every meal. It's advertised several times an hour on television. Grocery store aisles are full of practically nothing but starch. In fast-food restaurants, coffee shops, and convenience stores, there's little else to eat. If starch is a toxin, which it is if you're a diabetic or a prediabetic, you're definitely living in a toxic environment. Why is it so hard to avoid this stuff?

Let's go back to the Fertile Crescent. The ability to cultivate wheat gave prehistoric humans access to a larger and steadier source of calories than they had ever had. Because it allowed them to expand their numbers beyond that which could be supported by hunting game and gathering wild vegetation, they soon became dependent upon starch for their survival. It's understandable that they placed great value on the staples that kept them from starving. Our ancestors passed their reverence for these foods down through the generations. Europeans and Americans considered bread the mainstay of their existence—the "staff of life." In Judeo-Christian religious ceremonies, bread is a metaphor for life-giving sustenance. ("Give us today our daily bread.") The breaking and sharing of bread has been a symbol of friendship and unity for thousands of years. The consumption of wheat is so deeply entrenched in Western culture—as rice is in Eastern culture and corn is in Hispanic culture—that it's almost sacrilegious to suggest that these starches are responsible for epidemics of disease.

As for me, the more I learned about the "staff of life," the less I wanted to have anything to do with it and the more respect I gained for the diet of prehistoric humans. Meat and fresh vegetation have been part of the human diet for millions of years, while virtually all of the foods people eat that have high glycemic loads came after the advent of the Agricultural Age—many of them in the last hundred years. By eliminating flour products, potatoes, and rice, I was bringing my diet closer to the way humans ate for millions of years before they stumbled onto starch.

Cheap Calories

It didn't take long for our ancestors to figure out that land and labor used for growing starch could yield more calories than resources devoted to other crops. Wheat, potatoes, rice, and corn still provide far more calories with less investment of land, labor, and capital than any other foodstuff. Indeed, the United States has often had to deal with an *oversupply* of corn, wheat, and potatoes. For years, the American government paid farmers to reduce their production of those crops to prop up prices. In the 1970s, in response to rising food prices, the Department of Agriculture changed its policy and started encouraging farmers to produce as much food as they could. Production of corn, wheat, and potatoes skyrocketed, making starch cheaper and more abundant than ever.

The demand for goods usually drives supply, but occasionally supply generates demand. When corn farmers ended up with more corn than they could sell, they created a new market. They did what your digestive system does to starch: they converted it to sugar. They started marketing corn syrup as a cheap alternative to cane sugar. Now much of the corn Americans consume is in the form of a sweetener called *high-fructose corn syrup*. Indeed, because it's so cheap, corn syrup has replaced cane sugar as the main sweetener consumed by Americans.

The largest increase in sugar consumption in the United States in the past thirty years has been in sodas consumed mostly by kids. With a main ingredient as cheap as corn syrup, soda manufacturers could make drinks bigger with little added cost. Kids recognized a bargain and started buying pop in larger containers—twenty-ounce bottles and thirty-two-ounce containers. Economically, this was a win-win deal. Kids got more soda for their buck, and companies made more money. The downside was that skyrocketing sugar consumption contributed to an epidemic of childhood obesity and diabetes.

Oversupply of potatoes spurned a similar phenomenon. Instead of just selling whole, fresh potatoes, suppliers started slicing, pre-cooking, and freezing them and then selling them to fast-food restaurants as a labor-saving way to make french fries. Most of the increase in potato consumption in the past thirty years has been in french fries.

Because starch is cheap, the less money people have to spend on food, the starchier their diets tend to be. In many impoverished areas of the world, people eat little else but starch. They get enough calories from it, but without adequate meat and fresh vegetation, they often suffer from protein and vitamin deficiencies. Nutritional diseases, such as beriberi, scurvy, rickets, and iron deficiency anemia, are rampant in areas where people rely heavily on starches for calories.

In wealthier countries, most people can afford to eat enough protein and fresh vegetation to prevent vitamin deficiencies. Indeed, in terms of percentage of household income, food in the United States has never been cheaper. According to Department of Agriculture statistics, the average family in 2007 spent 9 percent of its income on food, compared with more than 20 percent in the 1950s and nearly 50 percent in the 1900s. Nevertheless, although most Americans could afford to eat higher-quality food, they still consume more calories as starch than in all other foods combined. Many of our eating habits arose from economic necessity during times when food was scarcer. People learned to save money by limiting the amount of meat, fresh fruit, and vegetables they ate and filling the void with starch. Bread, potatoes, and rice are the traditional "filler foods."

In the 1960s, the Department of Agriculture made the starchy, filler-food approach to diet into public policy with its "food pyramid," posters of which were displayed in schoolrooms throughout the country. Flour products, potatoes, and rice formed the largest part of the pyramid at the base; fruit and vegetables occupied the smaller middle section; and animal products—eggs, meat, and cheese—the smallest part at the tip. Although most people assumed the food pyramid represented the healthiest way to eat, it was actually developed in response to the problem of *under*-nutrition. Its purpose was to illustrate the *cheapest* way to eat without risking vitamin and protein deficiencies. Recently, the Department of Agriculture revised the food pyramid to reduce its emphasis on starches.

As I changed my diet, it became obvious to me and to my wife, who does the grocery shopping, that cutting out starch was going to cost us a little more at the grocery store. It's no coincidence that the lower the glycemic load of a food, the higher its price tends to be, but I was willing to pay it. I knew that the amount of money we would save skimping on food wouldn't pay for a month's worth of diabetes pills, let alone the financial burden of eye, kidney, or blood vessel damage.

When Others Are Buying the Groceries

If cutting out starch just meant spending more money at the grocery store, most Americans could afford to eat more fresh produce and less starch. Avoiding starch becomes more difficult, however, when someone else is paying for the ingredients of the food you eat. More than ever, Americans are eating food prepared by others—restaurant food, preprepared meals, and packaged food. Businesses that make their money preparing food for others profit more from feeding folks starch than they do from providing meat and fresh produce. That's why restaurants are happy to serve you bread before your meals. It reduces the amount of meat and fresh vegetables you will need to satisfy your hunger. Fast-food restaurants entice you with bargain burgers but make most of their money selling you french fries and soft drinks. In convenience stores, it's difficult to find any food that doesn't consist mainly of starch.

The Quest for Ever-Tastier Starch

When our ancestors first separated wheat from chaff, they couldn't have been very excited about its taste. Flour is essentially flavorless. (You can prove that to yourself by eating a spoonful of it.) For thousands of years, humans wracked their brains trying to figure out ways to make grain more appealing to eat. They ground it up, added water, and stuck it in hot sand to bake. They discovered that if they let the dough sit for a day or two, natural fermentation would create bubbles and make the bread fluffier. Over the centuries, they learned to add fat, yeast, sugar, salt, spices, bits of fruit, and chocolate and to bake it in different ways to improve the taste. Cooks perfected complex recipes for cookies, cakes, piecrusts, pancakes, chips, crackers, doughnuts, scones, bagels, and muffins. Finally, instead of being just a source of calories that could keep people from starving, wheat became a food they could really enjoy.

The incentive to come up with ever-tastier starch products skyrocketed when governments began granting companies patents for original recipes, which gave them exclusive rights to sell their products. Because flour products require unique combinations of ingredients and cooking procedures, it's easier to obtain patents on them than on other foods such as meat and fresh fruit and vegetables. Having exclusive rights to sell a product allows a company to charge whatever it thinks consumers will pay without worrying about other companies undercutting its price.

It's a different story for fresh produce. Meat and fresh fruit and vegetables require no processing, so there's no way to patent them. Producers can't exclude competition, because there are no unique recipes involved, and there is no way to distinguish fresh produce brought to market by one farmer from that of another.

The combination of cheap ingredients and high markups of price over costs, which patents allow, creates the potential for processed-food manufacturers to enjoy large profit margins. Indeed, companies that sell breakfast cereals, crackers, and soda—including General Mills, Nabisco, and Coca-Cola—are among the largest corporations in the world. Food manufacturers have an enormous incentive to come up with ever-tastier products made from cheap ingredients. Firms spend millions of dollars annually on research into new ways to get people to eat starch.

How Advertisers Influence Your Tastes in Food

Food manufacturers often go beyond providing what people want; they influence preferences through advertising. We're bombarded by commercials touting the health benefits of various breakfast cereals, telling us how much fun it is to drink sodas and reminding us how tasty chips and crackers are. Do you ever wonder why we rarely see television ads for meat or fresh fruit and vegetables?

To afford large advertising budgets, companies have to have money left over after paying the costs of producing their product. In other words, they have to sell their products at substantial markups of price over cost. The best way to do that is to use cheap ingredients and eliminate competition with patents—conditions ideally suited to starch-based, processed foods but not to fresh produce. You can't patent meat or fresh fruit and vegetables, so there's no way to exclude competition. Markets are highly competitive, which makes profit margins thin—too thin to afford much advertising.

One way marketers try to get you to buy their product is by taking advantage of your concerns about your health. Unfortunately, the messages are often misleading. When researchers discovered that soluble fiber—including the kind found in oats—lowers blood cholesterol levels slightly, the company that makes the oat-based cereal Cheerios began marketing that product as a way to reduce cholesterol. Actually, Cheerios doesn't contain enough soluble fiber to do much at all to cholesterol levels, and it is full of starch—a bad way to start the day if you have diabetes or prediabetes.

Some breakfast cereals advertise themselves as "heart healthy" because they contain whole grains and no cholesterol. However, there's no scientific evidence that any of them do anything that affects your heart except raise your blood sugar and damage the arteries that supply blood to it. (The U.S. Food and Drug Administration is now challenging the veracity of some of these claims.)

Animal rights and environmental groups have also gotten into the food propaganda game. There's no question that it would be kinder to other species and easier on the planet if humans ate more starch and fewer animal products. The problem is that humans weren't designed to eat that way. Eating healthily as a vegetarian requires more knowledge and commitment than just switching from meat to starch. Someday humans might find good substitutes for animal protein, but in the meantime, it's difficult to avoid animal products without filling the deficit with starch.

So if it sometimes feels as if the world is conspiring to get you to eat more starch, let's face it, it is. From your parents, who had to pay for the food you ate, to restaurants, convenience stores, purveyors of processed foods, environmentalists, and animal rights advocates, everyone benefits when you eat starch—*everyone but you*. What can you do about it? The first step is to see the world as it is. For the sake of economics rather than biological need, you have been coerced into eating a substance humans weren't designed to eat. Starch is a tasteless paste that has no nutritional value except to provide calories. It's a low-grade toxin that will raise your blood sugar, damage your arteries, and pickle whatever insulin-making cells you have left. If you think of it that way, flour products, potatoes, and rice aren't so appealing.

There's a cornucopia of delicious fresh produce at the grocery store at prices that are lower relative to other things we spend our money on than at any time in history. You will do yourself a favor by taking advantage of it.

Part 2

Six Steps to Optimal Control of Your Diabetes

Now you know what brings on type 2 diabetes. Physical inactivity combined with a genetic predisposition made your body insensitive to insulin. As a result, your insulin-making cells have had to make more insulin than normal to handle the carbohydrates in your diet. That wouldn't have been a problem if you ate mainly fat, protein, and fresh fruit and vegetables, but years of eating high-glycemic-load carbohydrates, like bread, potatoes, and rice, and drinking sugar-containing beverages have worn out your beta cells. You probably still make plenty of insulin, but not enough to keep your blood sugar down.

Although starch is instrumental in causing diabetes, it's not the only food that releases glucose into your bloodstream. Insulin resistance makes it difficult for your system to handle even good carbohydrates such as fresh fruit and vegetables. In addition, if you're like most people with type 2 diabetes, insulin resistance is throwing your good and bad cholesterol levels out of balance and raising your blood pressure, which are the last things you need, considering that high blood sugar makes your arteries especially vulnerable to damage from those problems.

To regain a healthy metabolism and prevent damage to eyes, kidneys, and blood vessels from type 2 diabetes, the first step is to reduce your starch intake. Then you need to eliminate persisting insulin resistance, correct any insulin deficit, and make sure your cholesterol and blood pressure are not just normal but better than normal. Part 2 gives you six steps to accomplish those objectives and achieve optimal control of your diabetes:

- **Purging starch from your diet** will show you how to reduce the glycemic load of your diet to a fraction of what it was by controlling the amount of starch you eat (Chapter 10).
- **Inhibiting starch absorption** will help you blunt the blood-sugar-raising effects of whatever starch is left in your diet by using strategies that block its passage into your bloodstream (Chapter 11).
- **Sensitizing your muscles to insulin** will show you how to relieve insulin resistance in your muscles, so your body can

better handle whatever glucose enters your bloodstream (Chapter 12).

- **Getting your liver to cooperate** will help you improve the way your liver handles glucose, which will lower your blood sugar and further reduce your body's requirements for insulin (Chapter 13).
- **Making up any insulin deficit with insulin** will help you determine when and how to add insulin to lower your blood sugar to normal and further reduce the strain on your insulin-making cells (Chapter 14).
- **Optimizing your cholesterol and blood pressure** will show you how to keep your diabetes from damaging your blood vessels by lowering your blood cholesterol and blood pressure (Chapter 15).

10

Step 1
Purging Starch from Your Diet

Reversing starch's harmful effects can be as simple as cutting out a few starchy foods that you might not like anyway. Flour products, potatoes, rice, corn, and sugar-containing soft drinks are the only commonly consumed foods that have glycemic loads greater than 100. If your diet is similar to the typical American diet and you eliminate those foods, you will lower the glycemic load of your diet to a fraction of what it was. Your diabetes will be easier to control, your body will start tapping into your fat stores for energy, and the insulin-driven tumor that is your belly will steadily shrink. You won't need to count calories, carbs, or fat grams. All you need to do is cut out those five foods. It really can be that simple.

The most important lesson to be learned from the glycemic-load measurements is that while some carbohydrates are good and some are bad, the bad ones aren't just a little worse than the others—they're terrible! The glycemic loads of typical servings of flour products, potatoes, rice, pasta, and most breakfast cereals are not just a little higher than those of natural carbohydrates like fresh fruit and vegetables—they're several times higher.

You should have no difficulty recognizing the culprits. One thing that makes eliminating starch easy is that it's rarely hidden or blended into other foods where you can't see it. It's always right out in the open. You can literally spot it from across the room. If you're not sure you can recognize starch when you see it, here's a list of common culprits:

White bread
Brown bread
White rice
Brown rice
Potatoes
Corn
Pasta
Breakfast cereals
Oatmeal
Pancakes
Bagels
English muffins
Cookies
Crackers
Potato chips
Corn bread

Get the picture? Anything that comes from grain, potatoes, rice, or corn.

It's Not the Sugar

Notice that sugar and candy are not on that list. That's because sugar is usually not a problem unless it's combined with starch. You might be thinking, "If I'm trying to avoid starch because it turns to sugar, why is it OK to eat sugar?" Here's why sugar and candy are not your enemies and can actually be your friends.

The glycemic loads of sugar and candy are lower than those of starches *because typical serving sizes are smaller.* It usually doesn't take much sugar or candy to satisfy most people's urge for something sweet. You don't need a pile of sugar the size of a potato to sweeten your coffee. The reason serving sizes in table sugar and candy are smaller is that you taste all of the glucose in them. Indeed, too much sweetness can be sickening. That's not true of bread, potatoes, or rice. The sugar molecules in starch are bonded to one another, which makes them unavailable to interact with your taste buds. You taste only about 2 percent of the sugar in starch. However, as soon as it hits your intestinal tract, it turns to pure sugar. As far as your blood glucose level is concerned, eating a baked potato is like eating a similar-size pile of sugar.

A modest serving of candy—say, a few squares of chocolate—shouldn't raise your blood sugar. However, it's a different story when you mix sugar with starch. Starch is highly absorbent. It dilutes the taste of anything you mix with it, so we tend to eat more sugar than we might otherwise when it's mixed with starch. Starchy sweets such as cookies, cakes, and pies are loaded with added sugar in addition to the sugar released by the breakdown of starch.

Whereas the glycemic loads of typical servings of bread, potatoes, or rice range between 250 and 350, the glycemic loads of many kinds of candy are comfortably less than 100. For example, a quarter-inch-thick, inch-square piece of dark chocolate has a glycemic load of approximately 25. A snack-size package of Peanut M&M's has a glycemic load of 43.

This is good news for those of us for whom dinner isn't complete without a taste of something sweet afterward.

What about ice cream? A scoop of ice cream—approximately a fourth of a cup—has a glycemic load of approximately 50, which is acceptable. The problem is that ice cream is basically a sugar-sweetened beverage—cream sweetened with sugar. Like a liquid, it slides over your tongue without interacting fully with your taste buds. In addition, freezing obscures the sweetness. Because you don't taste much of the sugar in ice cream, you need more of it to satisfy your craving for sweetness. Indeed, most folks don't stop at a fourth of a cup of ice cream.

Sugar at dessert should serve only to provide the sweetness you crave at the end of a meal, not to fill you up. After all, you just ate—you should already be full. You don't need another plateful of food. When you think of dessert, picture your cupped hand. That should be large enough to hold it.

It's best to avoid eating sugar or candy on an empty stomach. Other foods in your stomach help keep sugar from rushing into your bloodstream. Also, if you eat sweets when you're hungry, you'll tend to use them to quell your hunger rather than just to satisfy the urge for something sweet.

How Much Starch Can You Get Away With?

Although recognizing starch is easy, avoiding it can be logistically challenging. We're inundated by it. Dietary tradition dictates that a flour product, a potato, rice, or pasta be served with virtually every meal. Sometimes there's little else to eat. The reality is that some starch is probably going to pass your lips. Make no mistake, the most effective way to avoid the harm starch causes is to not eat it in the first place. However, if you have to eat some starch, even though you realize it causes nothing but trouble, it's helpful to know how much you can get away with.

Humans did not evolve to consume a carbohydrate-free diet. Although the glycemic load of the Paleolithic diet was much lower than ours, it wasn't zero. Our prehistoric ancestors ate some carbohydrate, just not enough to make them susceptible to diabetes and obesity. There is a "threshold" of glycemic load below which the risk of diabetes and heart disease is negligible. Studies of the relationships between glycemic load and disease indicate that the risk of diabetes and heart disease increases as *the daily sum of glycemic loads exceeds approximately 500*. It's no coincidence that this level of glycemic load also approximates the point below which overweight individuals usually lose weight, even if they are not trying to reduce calories. If you keep your daily glycemic load below approximately 500, your insulin levels will be low enough to allow calories to be mobilized from fat stores so you require less from your diet to satisfy your hunger.

Most truly "natural" foods—foods that are similar to ones that have been part of the human diet for millions of years—have glycemic loads less than 100. Most foods with glycemic loads greater than 100 are unnatural, processed foods—invariably a starch or a sugar-containing beverage. It's hard to go wrong if you stick to foods with glycemic loads less than 100. Indeed, if you abstain from starch and sugar-containing beverages completely, your daily glycemic load is unlikely to come anywhere near 500.

Actually, you can eat small amounts of starch and still stay below 500. Here's a rule of thumb that will allow you to have a little starch yet keep your daily glycemic load from exceeding 500:

Considering that a typical serving of bread, potatoes, rice, or pasta has a glycemic load of approximately 200 to 300 and the glycemic loads of the other foods you eat in a day typically add up to about 200 to 300, you can usually have *the equivalent of one typical serving of starch a day* without going much over 500. What's a "typical" serving? About as much as you can fit on a quarter of a regular-size plate. It's best to split this up—a half serving twice in a day, or a third of a serving three times in a day—and it should not be consumed on an empty stomach. Other foods will help prevent it from rushing into your bloodstream.

There's nothing inherently wrong with having a daily glycemic load *lower* than 500. You can do just fine eating no foods that break down to glucose. Your body can turn the protein and fat you eat into all the glucose it needs. Humans lived for millions of years with minuscule amounts of digestible carbohydrate in their diet. The trouble with trying to reduce your glycemic load too much is not that you need carbohydrate to stay healthy. The problem is food cravings. If you reduce your daily glycemic load below approximately 300 or so, you start having to eliminate foods you naturally crave—fresh fruits, vegetables, and sweets, and the odds are you won't keep it up for long. As America's experience with Atkins's radical low-carb diet taught us, food cravings usually win in the end.

One thing is for sure: it makes no sense to try to eliminate fruits and vegetables if you're still eating starch. One extra serving of starch will wipe out any gains you might make by reducing fresh fruit and vegetables.

Estimating Glycemic Load from Ingredient Lists on Packages

The labels of many packaged foods include the carbohydrate content in the nutrients list. Although knowing the carbohydrate content alone won't allow you to predict how much a food will raise blood sugar, you can estimate an *upper limit* of glycemic load— call it the worst-case scenario. For example, given that white bread gets absorbed into your bloodstream as fast as any other kind of food, if a snack contains less carbohydrate than a slice of white bread does, it can't raise your blood sugar more than a slice of white bread would. It might raise it less, but it can't raise it more.

The label usually lists how many grams of carbohydrate are in a typical serving and how much of that is fiber. If you subtract the grams of fiber from the total grams of carbohydrate, you come up with the "available" carbohydrate, the amount that goes into your bloodstream. Just remember the unlucky number *thirteen*. That's how many grams of available carbohydrate are in a slice of bread. If a serving of a food contains less than thirteen grams of available carbohydrate, even if it is absorbed as fast as white bread (worst-case scenario), it shouldn't raise your blood sugar more than a slice of bread would. In other words, its glycemic load should be less than 100, the glycemic load of a slice of white bread. For example, if a snack contains eight grams of carbohydrates and two of those grams are fiber, its available carbohydrate content is six grams. That's less than half the available carbohydrate in a slice of white bread, so its glycemic load should be less than half that of a slice of bread—less than 50. It might be a lot less or just a little less, but it has to be less than 50. You could have two servings of that snack and still stay under 100.

Measuring Your Own Glycemic Loads

For years, physicians monitored patients by measuring their blood sugar after they had fasted overnight. When home glucometers became available, doctors kept telling patients to measure their levels after fasting. It's a good idea to check your fasting blood sugar regularly to see how well you're managing your diabetes. However, once you have gotten your diabetes under reasonable control, you usually don't learn much from checking fasting levels all the time. You can generally predict what they're going to be. If you really want to get some useful information from your home measurements, get in the habit of checking your blood sugar *after* you've eaten. You can learn for yourself what various carbohydrates do to your blood sugar, and how exercise, medication, and other foods affect it. A reasonable goal is to keep your blood sugar two hours after eating from exceeding 160. If you keep your after-meal readings down, you're probably going to have good fasting levels.

The World's Easiest Diet

Of all the dietary strategies used to lose weight or treat diabetes, the easiest is to cut out starch. Starch is easy to recognize; you don't need a list of foods to tell you what to eat. It's essentially tasteless, so when you replace it with other foods, you actually increase the amount of flavor and variety in your diet. Starch contains no essential vitamins or minerals, so you avoid food cravings. It reduces your body's demands for insulin, which promotes weight loss and makes your blood sugar easier to control. Best of all, you usually don't have to consciously try to reduce the amout of food you eat.

If you have diabetes, there's nothing to be gained by worrying about dietary fat or cholesterol. As discussed in Chapter 4, low-fat, low-cholesterol diets have been a dead end. They don't reduce blood vessel disease or even lower blood cholesterol levels much. Nor do you need to worry about trans fats. Most of the trans fats in our food are in starches. All you need to do is cut out flour products, potatoes, rice, and sugar-containing liquids. That's as easy as it gets.

Here are some tips to help you get the starch out of your life:

- **Pick at your food.** Starch is usually separable from other foods. Use your fork to pick it out, and push it to one side of your plate.
- **Build a starch pile.** Try to eat the other things on your plate first, and put the starch in a pile on the side of your

plate. If you still feel like eating some starch after you've eaten everything else, go ahead and have a little. By that time, the other food has had a chance to reach your bloodstream. All that starch sitting in a heap won't look so good to you. When you leave the table, you can look at the starch pile and congratulate yourself on the glucose shock you avoided.

- **Combine meal-size salads with entrees.** Instead of the usual small salad before your lunch or dinner, have a meal-size salad with lots of hearty ingredients. Then skip the starchy side dishes and just go for the entree.

- **Don't start your day with a glucose shock.** The research has been done so many times that it's getting repetitive: if you have a starchy breakfast, your insulin levels will be higher, your blood sugar will fluctuate more, and you will tend to eat significantly more during the remainder of the day. If you must have some starch, try not to eat it for breakfast.

- **Learn to make a microwave omelet.** Some people say they don't have time to fix eggs for breakfast. You can make a microwave omelet in the time it takes to fix yourself a bowl of cereal. Just whip a couple of eggs and a glop of milk in a bowl and microwave it for three minutes at 40 percent power. Put a little butter, salt, and pepper on top, and you have a satisfying starchless breakfast.

- **Learn to make classic omelets.** I don't need to tell you how delicious a good omelet can be. I don't even need to tell you how to make one; instructions are all over the Internet. What I can tell you is that they're fun to cook and make a hearty breakfast that won't raise your blood sugar.

- **Eat All-Bran cereal regularly.** The modern diet is so refined that we have become grossly deficient in insoluble fiber. The only practical way to get enough of it to do you any good is to eat All-Bran cereal regularly. All-Bran cereal pushes the upper limits of glycemic load, so it's best to stick with a third of a cup but to eat it regularly.

A handful of chopped walnuts magically turns a bowl of bran cereal into a satisfying breakfast dish.

- **Learn to make a "wrap."** Sandwiches make it possible to eat lunch without a knife, fork, plate, and table. If you can't live without sandwiches, instead of putting the meat, lettuce, and mustard between two slices of bread (glycemic load 260), wrap them in a wheat tortilla. An eight-inch tortilla has a glycemic load of only 80—whole wheat ones, even less.

- **Try eating hamburgers bunless.** The only problem with hamburgers is the starchy bun. However, hamburgers are great without the bun. All that breading just gets in the way of the good stuff. You'll find that most restaurants are usually glad to comply. Put all the extras on it that you usually do, and eat it with a knife and fork. If you have to eat your burger with a bun, at least break away hunks of the upper bun as you eat it and put them in your starch pile.

- **Keep your glucometer where you will be two hours after eating.** Blood sugar measurements taken two hours after eating are invaluable. They'll tell you exactly what foods do to your blood sugar. However, it's easy to forget to check them. It helps to keep your glucometer close to where you usually are a couple hours after eating. Some glucometers have a beeper you can set to go off two hours after eating and a memory function that will keep track of fasting and after-meal readings separately.

11

Step 2
Inhibiting Starch Absorption

I t's easy to pass up bread, potatoes, and rice when they're side dishes, but occasionally starch is the main dish. There are probably going to be times when you can't avoid it. If you have to eat some starch, even though you know you shouldn't, there are some things you can do to lessen its blood-sugar-raising effects.

A concept that has fascinated weight-loss dieters for years is the notion of a "starch blocker," a supplement that would keep starch from entering the bloodstream. Then you could fill up on your favorite starches and still lose weight. If that sounds too good to be true, it is. No one has yet found a way to block starch from going into your system. The capacity of your digestive tract to extract every available calorie from your food is formidable. Keep in mind that for millions of years, survival of our species depended on the ability of our digestive tract to glean nutrition from whatever passed through it. The intestine evolved to be a powerful extractor of nutrients. Moreover, starch is the easiest of foods to digest. Your intestine is twenty-six feet long, but the first foot or two can absorb most of the starch you eat. If something is interfering with the absorption of starch, your digestive tract has plenty of time, copious amounts of enzymes, and a lot more intestine to finish the job.

However, while you can't stop starch from ultimately breaking down and entering your bloodstream, *you can slow down the process*. Indeed, the very concept of glycemic load is based on the fact that foods contain their own natural starch blockers. That's what keeps the glucose in vegetables from rushing into your bloodstream all at once. A large serving of broccoli might deliver as much glucose into your bloodstream as a slice of white bread, but it does so more slowly because it contains natural substances that interfere with the digestion of starch. If broccoli didn't contain those substances, its glycemic load would be the same as that of white bread. Indeed, you can take advantage of starch-blocking effects of foods you consume with starch to blunt starch's blood-sugar-raising effects. And yes, there are starch-blocking pills you can take that really work.

Natural Starch Blockers

The first line of defense against starch breaking down and rushing into your bloodstream is your stomach. Your stomach does not absorb food. Rather, it acts as a holding bin that regulates how fast food enters your intestine, where it is absorbed. Just having other foods in your stomach before eating starch reduces the blood sugar surge the starch would otherwise cause. Your stomach also acts as a mixing bowl, diluting starch with other foods, further slowing its absorption. Delaying the passage of starch into your intestines also gives the other nutrients you eat a chance to reach the appetite control centers in your brain, which helps prevent overeating.

Your intestine sends your stomach messages via nervous impulses and hormones, which govern the speed with which the stomach empties. When your intestine has all the food it can handle, it tells the stomach to stop allowing food to pass. Once the intestine has extracted all the calories it can and is ready for more food, it tells the stomach to let more pass. Type 2 diabetes often disturbs these messages and causes the stomach to empty too quickly. However, there are ways you can slow down stomach emptying so starch doesn't get absorbed so fast.

The makeup of the food mixture in the intestine determines the message the intestine sends to the stomach. Dietary fat in the intestine is a potent inhibitor of stomach emptying. A few bites of fatty food, such as nuts, cheese, or olives, ten or fifteen minutes before eating a starch-containing meal will reduce the resulting blood sugar surge. Nuts are especially effective. One study showed that a handful of nuts reduced the blood sugar surge from eating a helping of starch by 25 percent. A tablespoon of olive oil has a similar effect.

The fiber in fresh fruit and vegetables also slows the absorption of starch. Fiber is the indigestible part of fruit and vegetables. There are two kinds: soluble and insoluble. The insoluble kind is found in the husks and peels of fruit, vegetables, and grains. While insoluble fiber is essential for good colon health, that's not the kind of fiber that slows starch absorption. The other kind, soluble fiber, is found in the pulp of fruits and vegetables. In the intestine, it acts like a sponge, soaking up starch and slowing its absorption. Eating foods that contain soluble fiber—salad or fresh fruit and vegetables—with a meal helps blunt the blood-sugar-raising effects of starch.

In centuries past, vinegar was touted as a treatment for a variety of ills, including stomachaches, croup, heart failure, and poison ivy. Although most of those claims were baseless, researchers have discovered that a couple of tablespoons of vinegar taken with starch can reduce the resulting surge in blood sugar. Doctors used vinegar to treat diabetes for years before insulin became available. The active ingredient appears to be acetic acid. Although scientists aren't sure how vinegar works, they think acetic acid inhibits enzymes that digest starch. Apparently, it is not acidity per se that inhibits starch absorption, because other acids don't have the same effect.

High-protein foods such as eggs, dairy products, meat, and fish also reduce the blood sugar response to starch. Protein not only slows stomach emptying, but also enhances the insulin response.

Considering that nuts, olive oil, soluble fiber, vinegar, and protein all delay the absorption of starch, a hearty salad with olive oil dressing, vinegar, nuts, and cheese, eaten before a meal is bound to reduce after-meal blood sugar.

Actually, many of the foods we eat slow starch absorption. The effects are modest, usually not eliminating the surge completely—and they are no substitute for avoiding starch altogether—but the natural starch-blocking effects of fat, fiber, vinegar, and protein can keep a modest serving of starch from raising your blood sugar more than it would otherwise. The fact that so many foods interfere with its absorption tells us that starch consumed on an empty stomach is worse than starch eaten with other food.

Scientists have not systematically measured the starch-blocking effects of many foods. There's no glycemic load list of food combinations. That's where your glucometer comes in. You can measure your own blood sugar responses to various combinations of foods and to the order in which you eat them. You can learn for yourself if a particular food lessens the blood-sugar-raising effects of whatever starch you eat.

Starch-Blocking Pills That Work

In the 1980s, some diet supplement manufacturers claimed they had found a pill that could block the absorption of starch. It was an extract of white kidney beans called phaseolamin. In the test tube, it deactivated the enzyme responsible for breaking down starch to glucose. Advertisers touted it as a way to keep starch calories from entering the bloodstream and marketed it as a weight-loss product. Supposedly, it would allow dieters to continue enjoying their favorite starches and still lose weight.

It turned out phaseolamin was no match for the digestive powers of the human intestinal tract. When scientists studied its effects on humans, they found that it didn't keep starch from being absorbed at all. Unlike natural starch-blocking substances in low-glycemic-load foods, it didn't even slow absorption. Subsequently, the Food and Drug Administration banned companies from marketing the product as a weight-loss aid, and the whole notion of starch blockers fell into disrepute.

Although the idea that a person could take a pill to block the absorption of starch lost credibility with the public, medical scientists understood that the idea wasn't as unrealistic as it seemed. The breakdown of starch to glucose depends on the activity of a single enzyme, *amylase*, which breaks the bonds that holds the glucose molecules in starch together. Without amylase, your digestive tract can't absorb starch. Scientists knew that if they could find a way to deactivate amylase, they really could prevent starch from breaking down to glucose and entering the bloodstream.

In the 1990s, the pharmaceutical industry developed an effective amylase inhibitor called acarbose (pharmaceutical name Precose), which is currently available by doctor's prescription. It works by mimicking starch. Amylase tries to break acarbose down as it would starch, but acarbose ties up the enzyme and takes it out of action. Acarbose also slows down the absorption of sugar, although not as much as it does starch.

Like other starch blockers, acarbose is a poor match for the digestive powers of the human intestinal tract. It doesn't prevent starch from ultimately being broken down and absorbed into the bloodstream. What it does do, however, is delay the digestion of starch, essentially lowering its glycemic load. A dose of acarbose taken immediately before eating a serving of starch reduces the resulting blood glucose surge by up to 40 percent. For example, if the glycemic load of a slice of white bread is 100, a dose of acarbose can bring it down to approximately 60.

Like natural starch-blocking substances, acarbose only blunts the after-meal blood sugar spike; it doesn't reduce the amount that ultimately enters the bloodstream. The body still needs insulin to handle starch—just not as much as it would if all the glucose flooded into the bloodstream at once.

Acarbose is no substitute for avoiding starch. A very starchy meal can overwhelm its effects and cause an undesirable blood sugar surge. Nevertheless, if you have to eat some starch, a dose of acarbose taken immediately before the meal will reduce the starch's effect on your blood sugar and insulin levels.

Surprising Lessons from Acarbose

It could be argued that the reduced incidences of heart disease, diabetes, and obesity that researchers find among people who eat less starch are the result of factors other than eliminating after-meal blood sugar surges. Maybe it's just the high carbohydrate content of starch that causes trouble, not the fact that it gets absorbed faster than natural carbohydrates—the old "a carb is a carb" saw. Perhaps the vitamins and minerals in the foods that replace starch provide the benefit. Possibly something in the starchy foods we eat besides starch causes problems. Indeed, Americans consume most of the harmful trans fats they eat as amendments to starches. Acarbose gave scientists an ideal way to study the effects of reducing after-meal blood sugar surges without otherwise changing the diet. It provided some enlightening answers to these questions.

Several studies have found that taking acarbose before meals, without any other changes in the diet, not only reduces after-meal blood sugar and insulin levels, but also lowers blood triglyceride levels, decreases blood pressure, and promotes weight loss. In addition, it changes cholesterol particles from the small, dense kind associated with artery damage to the larger, lighter, less harmful type—just as avoiding dietary starch does. Indeed, acarbose substantially reduces the risk of heart attacks. In one study, researchers randomly assigned a group of patients with type 2 diabetes to take acarbose and compared their health over several years with that of a similar group of adult-onset diabetics who did not take acarbose. The heart attack rate in the group of patients taking acarbose was half that of the control group. Acarbose reduced the heart attack rate as much as any drug available for heart disease prevention today.

It's curious that while acarbose is popular in Europe, American doctors seem to have glossed over studies showing beneficial effects of acarbose on heart disease risk. Doctors, like everybody else, tend to see what they expect to see. They expected to see links between cholesterol and heart disease. They didn't expect to see links between after-meal blood sugar surges and heart disease.

Acarbose has been available for a couple of decades. Its patents expired before researchers discovered its benefits. Now it's so inexpensive that there's little profit to be made from selling it. Consequently, companies that manufacture acarbose don't advertise it as much as they do newer medications.

Acarbose is notably safe to take. Unlike most medications, it doesn't enter the bloodstream. It passes through the intestinal tract and into the colon, where it is broken down by bacteria. Allergic or toxic reactions are rare.

Acarbose has one common side effect: gassiness. Bacteria in your colon normally break down some of the food your intestine doesn't digest, and this often produces some gas. When starch that has been blocked from absorption in the intestine enters the colon, bacterial action often causes a temporary increase in gas production noticed the following day. This varies among individuals. Some people don't notice any increase at all; others find it intolerable. Gassiness usually decreases the longer you take acarbose. Most people don't mind some gassiness the next day if it means they can enjoy a favorite starch.

One reason acarbose isn't used as much as other diabetes medications is that doctors often assume that for maximum effectiveness, patients need to take it with every meal. That would be true if every meal contained starch. Hopefully, however, that won't apply to you, and there's no point in taking acarbose if you aren't about to eat some starch. You only need to take it with meals that contain enough starch to raise your blood sugar.

Another reason acarbose isn't as popular as other diabetes medications is that doctors and patients often focus on fasting blood sugar measurements and don't pay attention to after-meal levels. Acarbose doesn't have nearly as much effect on fasting levels as it does on after-meal levels, so its beneficial effects often are unappreciated.

My Pasta Pill

I know I should swear off pasta altogether. It would also be helpful if I refrained from eating the tortilla chips at my favorite Mexican restaurant. The occasional hamburger and french fries don't do me any good either. I've checked my blood sugar levels after these indiscretions, and as you would predict, they're awful.

I don't take acarbose regularly because I don't eat enough starch at most meals to raise my blood sugar. However, acarbose comes in handy for the lapses. I call it my "pasta pill." I keep a bottle of it in the kitchen for the occasional starchy meal. I also carry a couple of pills in my wallet in case I get stuck eating starch away from home. I've measured my blood sugar a couple of hours after taking acarbose with a starchy meal, and the levels, although not perfect, are usually reasonable.

Acarbose doesn't allow you to completely get away with eating a starchy meal. Your after-meal measurements will typically look better, but levels taken a few hours later might be a little higher than usual, reflecting the fact that acarbose doesn't block the absorption of starch, but just spreads it out over a longer period.

Although acarbose doesn't lower *fasting* blood sugar measurements by much, it lowers the overall average of blood sugar levels, encourages weight loss, and is remarkably effective at reducing the risk of diabetic complications. If you can't resist the occasional starchy meal, you might consider keeping a bottle of acarbose around to take before those lapses.

12

Step 3
Sensitizing Your Muscles to Insulin

I f you reduce the starch in your diet and do what you can to slow the absorption of whatever starch is left, your blood sugar levels will undoubtedly fall. However, even if your blood sugar comes down to normal, if you have type 2 diabetes or prediabetes, you have to realize that your body chemistry is still not normal. Your body is insensitive to insulin. It has to produce more insulin than normal to handle even good carbohydrates like fruit and vegetables. In addition, by the time you get type 2 diabetes, you've permanently lost about half of your insulin-producing beta cells. The remaining ones have to work overtime to make up for the ones that have been lost.

To keep what beta cells you have left from burning out, you need to reduce the strain on them as much as you can. The best way to do that is to reduce your body's demands for insulin not only by reducing the starch in your diet but also by increasing your body's sensitivity to the insulin you make.

129

Relieving insulin resistance not only makes your diabetes easier to control, it also promotes weight loss and helps keep your beta cells from burning out. In addition, it improves other conditions caused by insulin resistance, including high blood triglyceride, imbalances between good and bad cholesterol, polycystic ovary syndrome, and bothersome highs and lows of blood sugar.

The Critical Role of the Muscles in Type 2 Diabetes

Insulin resistance is not a problem with some internal organs such as your liver or kidneys. It's a *muscle* problem. Your muscles are your body's main glucose burners. They use fat and glucose for fuel to perform work. However, if they aren't doing much work, they don't need much fuel, so they stop responding to insulin.

Your muscles act like a computer that automatically switches to "sleep mode" to save electricity when not being used. If you don't use them for a day or two, they shut off to insulin. The good news is that, like a computer in sleep mode, they spring back to life when you use them again.

Everybody's muscles lose sensitivity to insulin when they're not being used. What's different about people who are genetically susceptible to insulin resistance is that their muscles go into a deeper-than-normal dormant state and become less responsive than normal to insulin when they aren't used. However, as soon as such folks exercise, their muscles spring back to life and start responding to insulin again, just like other people's muscles do.

The problem is that the muscles of modern humans spend too much time in that sleep mode. We aren't nearly as physically active as Mother Nature intended us to be. Although an increase in starch consumption in the last thirty years triggered an abrupt increase in the incidences of obesity and diabetes, the stage was set by declining levels of physical activity that started approximately a hundred years ago. There was much less obesity and diabetes then than there is now, but not because people ate less. Indeed, the average daily caloric intake was higher than it is now. What protected folks from obesity and diabetes in those days was that they were more physically active. Daily living generally required more physical activity than it does now. Mechanization hadn't taken over people's lives. Most Americans lived and worked on farms. Even city folks typically walked several miles a day just to get to work, and machines didn't do their work for them. They dug ditches, felled trees, and sawed lumber by hand.

Although we live in the Modern Age, the fact is that our bodies were made for the Stone Age. We simply weren't designed to be as sedentary as we are today. By reducing our muscles' sensitivity to insulin, the lack of physical activity that characterizes modern life makes us susceptible to obesity and diabetes.

The good news is that physical activity quickly *reverses* insulin resistance. But if you're thinking you're about to hear the same tired old advice to start sweating and straining, you're wrong. Exercise to relieve insulin resistance is different from other kinds of exercise. It's much easier. Truly, it can even be pleasant.

Targeting Exercise to Relieve Insulin Resistance

Different types of exercise achieve different goals. The kind of exercise that builds endurance is different from the kind that builds big muscles, and both of these kinds of exercise are different from the kind that improves insulin sensitivity. To understand why some kinds of exercise are better than others for relieving insulin resistance, it helps to know the difference between *aerobic* and *anaerobic* exercise.

Aerobic means "with air." *Anaerobic* means "without air." Aerobic exercise requires sustained repetitive movement, such as walking, running, cycling, or swimming. Anaerobic exercise involves straining against resistance for brief periods, such as in weight lifting. Both kinds of exercise require "air"—oxygen—to provide energy for the muscles that perform the work. The difference between anaerobic and aerobic exercise is in the timing. Aerobic exercise uses oxygen to provide energy *as the activity is taking place*; anaerobic exercise builds up an "oxygen debt," which is repaid *after exercise*. During aerobic exercise, oxygen-filled blood flows into the muscles steadily, refreshing their oxygen and allowing them to work continuously. During anaerobic exercise, muscles strain against resistance hard enough to squeeze off their blood supply. They have to work without oxygen. Blood refreshes their energy with oxygen during rest periods.

A hundred years ago, diabetes and obesity were less common not only among farmers but also among people who lived in cities. City people worked in stores and offices, just as we do. In those days, folks rarely exercised for the sake of exercise. Indeed, girls and women were discouraged from engaging in sweaty sports. Health clubs were nonexistent. Whatever exercise people did came as part of attending to their daily needs. So what did they do for exercise that we don't do?

Indeed, from the standpoint of physical exertion, life was different because there was much less motorized transportation. There were few cars, buses, elevators, or escalators. Trolleys and commuter trains serviced only a few routes in major cities. The main difference between the kinds of physical activity people did in the early twentieth century and what we do now is that *they walked more*. Even people with office jobs had to walk several miles a day to get to and from work and to perform their jobs.

Although walking may seem easy compared with other kinds of exercise, it turns out that it's remarkably effective at relieving insulin resistance. In a study of 73,743 women reported in the *New England Journal of Medicine*, researchers found that walking ten miles a week was as good for preventing diabetes and heart disease as working out at a gym three hours a week.

You might think there would be little point in walking for exercise if you were already working out at a gym regularly. However, this study found that walking ten miles a week in addition to exercising at a gym three hours a week reduced the risk of heart disease and diabetes considerably more than only exercising at a gym.

Other studies have shown that, for preventing diabetes, the difference between walking just twenty minutes four days a week and not doing any exercise at all is greater than the difference between long-distance running and walking. What this means is not just that walking is good for you—you already knew that—it's that lack of any exercise at all is *terrible* for you. If you aren't at least walking twenty minutes every other day, you're a sick puppy! You're in a metabolically deranged state that makes you prone to diabetes, heart disease, obesity, and infertility.

"No Pain" Doesn't Mean "No Gain"

Considering how easy walking is, compared with other kinds of exercise, you might wonder why it's so effective at preventing diabetes. The answer lies in tiny energy-producing units in muscle cells called *mitochondria*. These little dynamos use oxygen to burn fuel, which produces energy for muscle cells to do their work. Scientists have found that the mitochondria of people with insulin resistance are less active than normal. In fact, people with family histories of type 2 diabetes have this quirk long before they develop any other signs of diabetes.

As it turns out, most of the mitochondria in your body are in your walking muscles, which explains why regular walking is so effective at restoring insulin sensitivity and preventing diabetes. Your mitochondria are where the problem is if you have insulin resistance, and walking activates them, which makes your muscles respond to insulin.

It might seem hard to believe that something as undemanding as walking could do you so much good. No pain, no gain, right? You might find it hard to believe, but the fact is that some muscles don't get tired when you exercise them. If you have trouble believing that, consider your diaphragm, the breathing muscle below your rib cage. How much effort does it take to breathe? That muscle works tirelessly day in, day out without producing any sense of fatigue at all. In fact, you're not even aware that it's working.

The reason your diaphragm never fatigues has to do with the kind of muscles that power it. Your body has two distinct kinds of muscle fibers, type 1 and type 2. You use your type 2 fibers for anaerobic exercise—activities that require brief exertion against resistance such as weight lifting. Because these fibers don't use much oxygen as they are being used, they contain only a few mitochondria. Instead, they incur an oxygen debt, which is repaid during rest, and it's that oxygen debt that creates the sense of fatigue.

As the deficit builds, fatigue increases until you rest and repay the debt.

Type 1 fibers work differently. Because they specialize in steady, repetitive work, they are richly endowed with mitochondria. This allows them to use oxygen to replenish energy as they are being used. Because they don't incur an oxygen debt, they don't get fatigued.

The reason your diaphragm can work continuously without fatigue is that it's powered by the those untiring type 1 muscle fibers. The large numbers of mitochondria in these fibers restore the energy in the muscles as they are working, which keeps them from building up an oxygen debt and becoming fatigued.

But what does your diaphragm have to do with walking? All creatures must do two things to survive: breathe and get from one place to another. Mother Nature made sure the muscles that do these jobs could work without getting fatigued, so she powered them with those untiring type 1 fibers. Although your diaphragm accounts for only a small portion of your total muscle mass, your walking muscles are another matter. They make up about 70 percent of your muscle mass, and like your diaphragm, they're powered by type 1 muscle fibers.

There's the beauty of it. The very kind of muscle activity that restores insulin sensitivity the most is exactly the kind that produces the least fatigue.

Try this experiment on yourself. As you're walking, increase your speed until you feel the muscles in your legs start to get tired. Then gradually slow down. You'll find that you only have to slow down a little before the fatigue in your legs abruptly disappears. That's the point at which your mitochondria are completely replenishing the energy your muscles are using. You're no longer accumulating an oxygen debt. It's your natural walking speed. At that speed, you could walk for hours. You might get bored, your feet might get sore, but muscle fatigue would not be a problem. What other exercise could you do continuously for hours without being limited by muscle fatigue?

As easy as walking is, you're actually expending more energy than you think. Scientists can measure the amount of energy muscles expend in exercise. They also have a scale for rating the amount of fatigue people experience during exertion. They have found that of all the common kinds of exercise people do, walking activates the most mitochondria with by far the least sense of fatigue.

Even though exercise burns calories, the benefit you derive from it is not simply a matter of expending calories. Indeed, most folks are surprised to find out how few calories are burned off by even the most vigorous exercise. For example, you would have to run ten miles to burn off the calories provided by a typical dinner. Exercise promotes weight loss and prevents diabetes not because it burns off calories but because *it increases the body's sensitivity to insulin.*

How Much Exercise Does It Take?

Your muscles' sensitivity to insulin behaves like a switch. It's largely either on or off. Walking a couple of miles turns it on. Sitting all day turns it off. Walking more than a couple of miles increases insulin sensitivity further, but not as much as you might expect. You get the most benefit out of the first two miles.

Similarly, running a couple of miles instead of walking increases insulin sensitivity further, but not as much as you might think. The important thing is to go the distance. Walking a couple of miles is almost as good as running the same distance.

What about other kinds of exercise? If you want to build big muscles, you need to strain against resistance, as you do when you lift weights. The no-pain-no-gain rule applies. If you want to compete in a ten-kilometer footrace, you need to increase the amount of blood your heart can pump by pushing yourself toward the point of exhaustion. The no-pain-no-gain rule applies there, too. But if all you want to do is wake up the mitochondria in your type 1 muscle fibers and relieve insulin resistance, all you need to do is walk. The no-pain-no-gain rule does not apply. You can walk farther or run if you want, but the effect on insulin resistance is not much greater. The advantage of walking over running is that it's much easier. You might even find it pleasant.

Here's the catch. When it comes to losing weight and treating or preventing diabetes, it's not the intensity of exercise that counts, *it's the regularity.* It doesn't matter whether you run a marathon or walk a couple of miles; the effect on your muscles' sensitivity to insulin dwindles away in twenty-four to forty-eight hours. To keep insulin resistance at bay, you need to exercise at least every other day. If you're just a weekend exerciser, by Tuesday your muscles are back in sleep mode. Your body will spend the next four days in an insulin-resistant, obesity-promoting state.

A Good Addiction

Every working day of my life, I talk to people about their exercise habits. Most folks know they would be healthier if they exercised, but they just never get around to doing it. The usual excuse is that they don't have time, but I know that's not true. Many of the busiest people find time to exercise, and a lot of folks with plenty of time on their hands think they're too busy. If you have time to watch a half hour of television, you have time to walk enough to restore your body's sensitivity to insulin.

It's really not lack of time that keeps people from exercising. Exercise requires physical exertion, and the reality is that humans are naturally averse to physical exertion. The problem is we're naturally lazy. It's a survival mechanism. Cave dwellers had no business leaving their caves if they didn't need to. It just burned energy and increased their chances of being eaten by a large animal.

However, we couldn't sit in our caves too long. We needed to get out and track down some food. Mother Nature made sure that once our prehistoric ancestors left their lairs and got into the hunt, their attitudes changed—they became energized. Exercise raises the level of natural mood enhancers in your nervous system just as antidepressant medications do. Studies show that walking programs relieve mild depression as effectively as medication. Exercise also stimulates *endorphins*, the body's natural painkillers, which relieve aches and pains and promote a feeling of calmness and well-being. It also raises your level of adrenaline, which gives you energy and strength.

Antidepressant? Painkiller? Tranquilizer? Energizer? If exercise were a drug, you couldn't keep people away from it! Exercise—like religious conversion, falling in love, or kicking a harmful addiction—changes people's lives. It's no wonder some people are addicted to it.

Every year, thousands of people join health clubs they never attend and buy exercise equipment they never use. The idea of exercising sounds great right up until it's time to do it. That's when the aversion strikes. It happens to all of us. A wave of lethargy comes over you, and exercise doesn't sound so good after all.

The challenge is to overcome your natural aversion to exercise. If you ask any regular exerciser, he or she tell you that the trick is to take the first step. You might feel sluggish and averse to the idea of exerting yourself while you're sitting on your couch, but once you get halfway down the block, you find that your attitude changes.

Many people assume that the point of exercise is to sweat and strain. They think exercising means working out at a gym or running for miles. Although the rewards of strenuous exercise are great, such exercise requires too much effort for most people to do dependably and regularly. Any middle-aged person or older who tells you that working out at a gym or running long distances is pleasant is probably being disingenuous. It takes a special kind of motivation to do it—motivation a lot of us don't have. And that's where walking comes in. Of all the exercises you can do to improve your health, walking will give you the most benefit with the least effort.

Returning to the Nineteenth Century— Physically

As a doctor, knowing from experience what diabetes could do to my eyes, kidneys, and blood vessels was like someone holding a gun to my head and telling me to change my ways. Actually, I worked out at a gym before I got diabetes. However, my exercise habits weren't ideal for managing my diabetes. I exercised intensely but sporadically, and often I would get distracted and go for days without exercising. In other words, I spent too much time in an insulin-resistant state.

Once I understood that the best kind of exercise for diabetes was not so much a matter of intensity as regularity—and that for restoring insulin sensitivity, walking was almost as effective as more intense exercise—I changed my approach and started walking more.

One day I saw a photograph in the *Seattle Times* of a group of office workers taken in 1915. They were all slim and trim. It dawned on me that the only physical activity they did that I didn't do was walk to work. Most of the residential neighborhoods in Seattle were more than a mile from the business district. People who worked downtown had to walk at least a couple of miles a day to get to and from work.

That photograph inspired me. It was early summer, and the weather was pleasant, so I decided to leave my car at home and walk to work, just to see what it was like. I was surprised at how pleasant it was. That was five years ago. I never stopped. I gave up my pricey downtown parking space and have been walking two and a half miles to and from work ever since.

I have little doubt that my walking program has had a beneficial effect on my diabetes. Most people with diabetes need more medication as the years pass, but I'm actually using the same now as I did ten years ago. Many diabetics continue to gain weight. I've made no effort to cut calories, but I'm twenty-five pounds lighter than I was then. If for some reason I go for a day without exercise, I can immediately see the effects on my blood sugar. If I am walking regularly, I can usually get away with a small serving of starch with dinner and maybe a little dessert afterward. If I don't exercise, my after-meal blood sugar levels increase enough to make the difference between good and poor control of diabetes.

How Much, How Often, and When?

Dozens of research studies have shown that all it takes is thirty minutes of brisk walking to restore the body's sensitivity to insulin. Walking longer provides a little added benefit, but not nearly as much the first thirty minutes.

How fast should you go? You don't need to make yourself uncomfortable—you should be able to talk as you walk—but you shouldn't dawdle either. You should walk as if you had an appointment to keep—like a nineteenth-century person walking to work.

No matter how long or hard you exercise, insulin sensitivity begins to dwindle after twenty-four hours and is gone by forty-eight. Whatever you do, you need to do it at least every other day. That's why the National Institutes of Health recommends thirty minutes of exercise, four days a week. If you have type 2 diabetes, considering that insulin resistance played a large role in bringing it on, you would be smart to do more than that—maybe forty-five minutes—and do it every day.

One common misconception many diabetics have is thinking they have to exercise after meals to burn off the calories they just ate. That's certainly better than not exercising at all, but it actually works better to exercise in the hours before a starch-containing meal. The objective is not to burn off glucose that builds up in your blood but rather to sensitize your body to insulin to keep glucose from building up in your blood in the first place.

Light activities such as walking across the office to the water-cooler or cooking dinner don't qualify as exercise. Nevertheless, scientists have discovered that the small movements people make throughout the day add up to have an important effect on body chemistry. They call it the "fidget factor," and it strongly influences people's tendency to gain weight. Among activities that have the lowest fidget factors are those that involve watching a screen, such as working at a computer or watching television. Computers and television mesmerize people, freezing their body movements. The more time people spend in front of a computer or watching television, the more problems they have with weight gain. If you work at a computer all day, watch television at night, *and* don't exercise, you're bound to have trouble controlling your diabetes and your weight. In a study reported in the *New England Journal of Medicine* in 2002, researchers found that sitting more than twelve hours a day increases the risk of heart disease by 40 percent. If your job requires you to spend hours in front of a computer, daily exercise is a must.

The Benefits of Other Kinds of Exercise

If you have type 2 diabetes or prediabetes, the most important thing aerobic exercise can do for you is to restore insulin sensitivity, and as discussed, to do that, it doesn't have to be intense. It just has to continue steadily for thirty minutes or so. That is not to say that more intense exercise, like running, isn't beneficial. Pushing your oxygen-consuming type 1 fibers further toward the point of fatigue requires that the heart pump more blood, which strengthens the heart muscle, improves endurance, and promotes changes in arteries that allow them to carry more blood.

We all know the heart is important, but you might wonder why you need to strengthen the heart muscle and have great endurance. Indeed, unless you're planning to compete in a footrace, you really don't need an exceptionally strong heart muscle or outstanding endurance. To control diabetes and lose weight, all you need to do is restore your body's sensitivity to insulin, and you can do that by just walking.

Because the muscles that perform anaerobic or "resistive" exercise such as weight lifting consist mainly of type 2 muscle fibers, which don't contain many mitochondria, exercising them doesn't restore insulin sensitivity as well as aerobic exercise does. However, anaerobic exercise is superior to aerobic exercise for increasing muscle strength and size. All muscles respond to insulin, so the larger your muscle mass, the more sensitive you are to insulin. Also, the more muscle you have, the more calories you burn—not just when you're exercising but also while you're at rest. Indeed, weight training adds to the insulin-sensitizing benefits of aerobic exercise. In a study reported in the journal *Diabetes Care* in 2003, researchers assigned one group of adult-onset diabetics to an aerobic exercise program and compared their insulin sensitivity with another group assigned to the same program but with fifteen minutes of resistive exercises added to each exercise session. After four months, the insulin sensitivity of the patients who added resistance exercise to their exercise program was higher than that of the ones who did aerobic exercise alone.

Anaerobic exercise requires some straining, which most people consider harder than walking. The good news is that you only have to do it for a few minutes a couple of times a week to build muscle strength and mass. Scientists who study exercise found that the optimum strengthening routine for a muscle group is two sets of ten repetitions, with the second set being against maximal resistance.

Resistance exercise can help you in another way. Losing weight too fast reduces your muscle mass, which slows your metabolism and makes further weight loss more difficult. This reduction in the rate at which you burn off calories starts in the first couple of weeks and persists for months, virtually guaranteeing that the lost weight will come back. Indeed, diet-induced metabolic slowdown is the nemesis of all strict diets, but here's the worst of it. Diet-induced metabolic slowdown sticks around for months after you've regained the weight you lost, which makes you gain even more weight. In other words, strict low-calorie diets can ultimately make you gain weight.

The best way to avoid diet-induced metabolic slowdown is to avoid losing weight too fast—a couple of pounds a month is fine. However, by preserving your muscle mass, resistance exercise prevents diet-induced metabolic slowdown.

Resistance exercise is one of the best things you can do to stave off some of the objectionable effects of aging. As we get older, we tend to lose muscle mass, a process that accelerates after age forty. In women, the loss of estrogen that occurs around menopause accelerates this decline. Age-related muscle loss contributes heavily to the tendency for men and women to develop insulin resistance as they age. Indeed, between ages twenty and sixty, the incidence of insulin resistance almost doubles. Weight training can prevent much of the loss of muscle mass and insulin sensitivity that aging and menopause bring on.

Crafting an Ideal Exercise Program

If you consider the benefits of anaerobic and aerobic exercise, you can understand why people who exercise regularly feel better, live longer, and have more active lives than couch potatoes do. As a doctor who had seen the consequences of poorly controlled diabetes, I knew I had to get serious about exercise. I also knew I needed to be realistic about the limits of my own willpower. I developed an exercise pattern that not only maintains insulin sensitivity but also provides the benefits of endurance and strength training. It's also a program that my limited willpower and schedule allow me to do.

To stay sensitive to insulin, I make a point of doing at least a half hour of aerobic exercise every day, either walking or using an elliptical trainer. To maintain cardiovascular endurance and muscle strength, I go to a gym twice a week and do intense aerobic exercise and weight training. Every muscle contributes to the body's metabolic activity, so I try to strengthen all major muscle groups. I use exercise equipment to flex and extend every joint against resistance. That amounts to about fifteen different exercises.

Around age fifty, I began to find that jogging was jarring on my bones and ligaments. Elliptical trainers and StairMasters are ideal substitutes for running because they're easy on the joints.

If any part of my exercise program contributed to the twenty-five pounds of weight I have lost in the past ten years, it would have been the added walking. I was working out at a gym a couple of times a week *before* I got diabetes. The only difference now is that I walk on days I don't go to the gym.

13

Step 4

Getting Your Liver
to Cooperate

A couple of weeks after I discovered that I had diabetes, my fasting blood sugar had come down to around 160—much better than 380, where it started, but still not normal. If I had given my low-carbohydrate diet and exercise program more time to work, my blood sugar probably would have come down further, but I started taking medication anyway. You might ask why, if type 2 diabetes is so dependent on lifestyle, I didn't try to control it with diet and exercise alone. Why was I so quick to take medication?

It's true that the combination of too much starch and not enough exercise brings on diabetes, and you can improve it a lot by eating right and restoring your body's sensitivity to insulin with exercise. However, even if you get your blood sugar back down to normal, your body's capacity to deal with carbohydrates is never the same. Your beta cells never regain their normal ability to produce insulin.

Diabetes doesn't start the day your blood sugar goes up. For years beforehand, your body has difficulty handling foods that break down to glucose. During this "prediabetic" phase, your beta cells make plenty of insulin, but because your muscles lose sensitivity to it, you have to make as much as five or six times the normal amount of insulin to handle the carbohydrates in your diet. Consequently, your beta cells virtually wear out from overwork. By the time your fasting blood sugar rises, your body has lost about half of its normal capacity to produce insulin. Even if you correct the problems that brought on your diabetes, you can't bring all of those lost beta cells back.

The reason I was happy to take medication was not just that it could lower my blood sugar—I probably could have brought my levels down further without pills—but because it would relieve some of the burden on my beta cells and keep them from burning out. I realized that the ability of my beta cells to make insulin would never return to normal, but I knew that reducing demands on them would forestall further damage and maybe even restore some of their function.

Your Uncooperative Liver

Although eliminating dietary starch and restoring your muscles' sensitivity to insulin will improve your diabetes greatly, for your body to handle glucose normally you have to deal with another problem: an uncooperative liver.

One of your liver's jobs is to guard against low blood sugar. It stores up glucose for release back into the bloodstream should the glucose level in your blood get too low. One of insulin's jobs is to regulate the ebb and flow of glucose in and out of your liver. Normally, when your blood sugar rises, your beta cells produce more insulin, which drives glucose into your liver. When your blood sugar falls, your beta cells produce less insulin, which allows the liver to release glucose back into your bloodstream if necessary. When your beta cells start wearing out, the coordination between them and your liver goes awry. Your liver releases glucose into your bloodstream at inappropriate times, even when your blood sugar is high. This has the same effect as eating more starch, so even though you're doing your best to avoid starch, your liver works against you.

Whereas cutting out starch will reduce the amount of glucose entering your bloodstream and exercise will restore your muscles' sensitivity to insulin, once you damage your beta cells, the normal coordination between your liver and your beta cells is lost. Your liver will continue to release glucose into your bloodstream at inappropriate times, which increases your body's demands for insulin. The only way to get your liver to cooperate is to take medication. Indeed, some of the most effective medications for treating type 2 diabetes are ones that keep the liver from secreting glucose into the bloodstream when it shouldn't.

Liver Sensitizers

In the early 1990s, the pharmaceutical company Bristol-Meyers Squibb introduced a new diabetes medication called metformin (trade name Glucophage). Metformin is derived from French lilac, an herb used for centuries for treating diabetes. Whereas the pills that doctors had been using previously worked by spurring beta cells to make more insulin, metformin worked differently. By keeping the liver from pouring glucose into the bloodstream when it shouldn't, it reduced the body's requirements for insulin.

Like many breakthroughs in medicine, metformin's potential wasn't appreciated at first. Most doctors didn't understand the importance of improving insulin sensitivity in treating adult-onset diabetes. They thought adult-onset diabetes was just a milder form of the kind kids got—a problem of insulin deficiency. Because metformin did nothing to increase insulin production, most doctors regarded metformin as a poor substitute for the older drugs.

Because metformin keeps the liver from pouring glucose into the bloodstream, it reduces the amount of insulin the beta cells have to make to keep the blood sugar down. By reducing the burden on the beta cells—or at least by not spurring them to produce more insulin, as the older pills do—metformin helps keep them from wearing out.

Most remarkable, however, is metformin's effectiveness at preventing the long-term complications of diabetes. Metformin helps prevent not only microvascular injury (damage to the tiny vessels in the eye, kidney, and nerves), but also macrovascular damage

(damage to large blood vessels), which causes heart attacks and strokes. Excessive insulin production increases the risk of heart attack and stroke even in the absence of diabetes. It is not surprising that reducing the body's insulin needs with metformin reduces the risk of those complications.

Although several other medications are now available that reduce the body's insulin requirements, metformin has the longest and best record for preventing the complications of diabetes. In 2008, the *New England Journal of Medicine* reported the results of a study of several thousands of patients with type 2 diabetes, who were tracked for seventeen years. Treatment with metformin reduced the heart attack rate by 44 percent. No other diabetes medication has been as effective as metformin for reducing the risk of heart attacks and strokes in patients with adult diabetes.

Before metformin became available in the early 1990s, the pills doctors had been prescribing, called *sulfonylureas*, worked by pushing the beta cells to make more insulin. Most doctors didn't realize that because of the body's lack of sensitivity to insulin, those cells were already producing more than normal amounts of insulin. Although sulfonylureas worked OK for lowering blood sugar at first, as the beta cells wore out, the pills became less effective. It was like whipping a tired horse. Recent studies have shown that beta cells burn out sooner among patients who take sulfonylureas than among patients using insulin-sensitizing medication like metformin.

Sulfonylureas had another objectionable side effect: by increasing insulin levels that were already too high, they made patients gain weight. However, doctors usually didn't worry much about that. They figured weight gain was a sign of improving health rather than a manifestation of excessive insulin production.

In contrast to sufonylureas, metformin does not cause weight gain. In fact, because it reduces the body's need for insulin, it often causes mild weight loss. Metformin is especially good treatment for overweight patients with diabetes. In a large study reported in the *New England Journal of Medicine* in 2008 comparing the effects of different treatments of type 2 diabetes, metformin was particularly effective for preventing heart attacks and strokes among overweight patients.

The Sooner You Start Metformin, the Better

Researchers have found that the sooner metformin is started, the more effective it is at preventing the complications of diabetes. This brings up a question: if insulin resistance goes on for years before your blood sugar levels rise, why wait for your doctor to tell you that you have diabetes before taking metformin? Why not take the pressure off your beta cells earlier and try to prevent them from wearing out? Indeed, several studies have shown that metformin can prevent or forestall diabetes in people with insulin resistance and prediabetes.

In addition to lowering blood sugar, metformin improves the balance between good and bad cholesterol, lowers blood pressure, and is effective treatment for polycystic ovary syndrome—all conditions associated with insulin resistance. Because metformin reduces the body's demands for insulin and forestalls beta cell failure, I encourage patients with type 2 diabetes to take metformin even if they are able to control their blood sugar levels with diet and exercise alone.

Physicians rarely prescribe metformin to patients who don't have diabetes, because they don't consider insulin resistance a disease. They have a point. Approximately 22 percent of the American population—44 percent of persons older than fifty—have insulin resistance. It's hard to accept that nearly half the American population have a disease. However, some doctors are starting to prescribe metformin to people who have insulin resistance without diabetes. I sometimes prescribe it for overweight patients who I am convinced are at unusually high risk of developing diabetes or for women who have polycystic ovary syndrome.

Most people who take metformin have no noticeable side effects. Most of the metformin in an oral dose gets absorbed in the upper part of the intestinal tract, but occasionally some of it gets through to the colon, where it can irritate the colon's lining and cause diarrhea. This is generally harmless, but it can be annoying. Taking metformin with food delays its passage through the intestinal tract, which sometimes helps. Pharmaceutical companies have recently reengineered metformin tablets to slow their passage through the digestive tract. By keeping the drug from reaching the colon, this formulation is less likely to cause diarrhea.

A rare but serious side effect of metformin is acidosis, a buildup of acid in the blood. This occurs predominantly in patients who have sluggish kidneys. Although metformin does not damage the kidneys, it leaves the body through the urine, so if the kidneys don't work normally, metformin can build up in the bloodstream. It's advisable to have a blood test to make sure your kidneys work OK before taking metformin.

To get the most benefit from metformin, doctors usually try to increase the dosage to its maximum, about 2,000 milligrams per day. Taking more provides little added benefit. If the maximal dose causes side effects, you can still benefit from a smaller dose. Even 500 milligrams a day helps.

Other Liver Sensitizers

In the past few years, pharmaceutical companies have developed several other drugs that keep the liver from spilling glucose into the bloodstream when it shouldn't. The first of these newer drugs is a type of medication called a TZD. The two currently available TZDs are rosiglitazone (trade name Avandia) and pioglitazone (trade name Actos). In addition to sensitizing the liver to insulin, TZDs have a slight muscle-sensitizing effect. Unlike metformin, they don't cause diarrhea. However, they often cause weight gain, which, though always unwelcome, is usually mild. TZDs can also cause fluid retention, which can be detrimental to patients with congestive heart failure.

Recently, pharmaceutical companies introduced a new class of medication that inhibits the action of *glucagon*, a hormone that causes the liver to release glucose into the bloodstream. Diabetics often make too much glucagon. Glucagon inhibitors keep the liver from releasing glucose into the bloodstream when it shouldn't and reduce the body's demands for insulin, just as metformin and TZDs do. Drugs of this type include exenatide (trade name Byetta), sitagliptin (trade name Januvia), amylin (trade name Symlin), and saxaglyptin (trade name Onglyza). These newer drugs are good alternatives for patients who can't take metformin because of side effects or concerns about poor kidney function. However, they all work better when combined with metformin.

Exenatide is especially useful for overweight patients with type 2 diabetes. It mimics the actions of a natural hormone in your body called incretin, which is deficient in type 2 diabetes. Exenatide not only lowers blood sugar but also slows digestion and promotes weight loss. In thirty years of practicing medicine, I have never seen a drug that could reliably produce long-term weight loss until exenatide came along. It promotes steady, lasting weight loss in overweight type 2 diabetics, especially if combined with metformin. The main objection patients have to exenatide is that it has to be administered by injection. However, once they get over their squeamishness about giving themselves shots and see the effects exenatide has on their weight and blood sugar, they're usually happy to take it.

Table 13.1 lists the medications commonly used today for type 2 diabetes.

Shortly before I discovered my diabetes, a large study showed that metformin prevents not only the microvascular complications of diabetes—eye, kidney, and nerve damage—but also the macro-vascular complications such as heart attacks and strokes, which is why I chose to take it. I figured anything that reduces my body's demands for insulin would take the pressure off my beta cells and help keep them from wearing out.

Maybe I figured right. Most doctors consider it inevitable that diabetics need stronger doses of medication with each passing year. That has not been true for me. I'm taking the same dosages of medication that I did ten years ago.

Table 13.1 **Popular Medications for Type 2 Diabetes**

Name (Trade Name)	Action	Advantages	Disadvantages	Comment
Starch Blockers				
Acarbose (Precose)	Inhibits enzyme that breaks down starch into glucose	Reduces after-meal blood sugar levels; prevents heart attacks; inexpensive	Can cause flatulence	Only needs to be taken before starchy meals; probably the safest of all diabetes medications
Insulin Sensitizers				
Metformin (Glucophage, Glumetza)	Prevents liver from releasing glucose into bloodstream	Improves insulin resistance; reduces insulin needs; preserves beta cells; promotes weight loss; prevents heart attacks; inexpensive	Can cause diarrhea; rarely causes dangerous acidosis in patients with kidney failure	Generally considered the first drug of choice for type 2 diabetes
Pioglitazone (Actos); rosiglitazone (Avandia)	Prevents liver from releasing glucose into bloodstream; increases muscle sensitivity to insulin	Improves insulin resistance; reduces insulin needs; preserves beta cells	Causes mild weight gain and fluid retention; sometimes worsens congestive heart failure; expensive	Often used as an alternative to metformin
Exenatide (Byetta)	Prevents liver from releasing glucose; increases insulin output from beta cells; slows stomach emptying	Causes significant weight loss, especially when combined with metformin	Must be taken by injection before meals; serious side effects are rare; expensive	Probably the most effective medication for losing weight ever developed; increasingly used as first drug of choice after metformin in overweight patients

Sitagliptin (Januvia)	Works like exenatide	Promotes weight loss; can be taken orally once a day	Not as good as exenatide for losing weight; serious side effects are rare; expensive	A good alternative to exenatide when injections are impractical
Amylin (Symlin)	Prevents liver from releasing glucose into bloodstream; slows stomach emptying	Promotes weight loss	Must be taken by injection before meals; not as good as exenatide for losing weight; expensive	Used as an alternative to exenatide
Beta Cell Stimulators				
Glyburide	Spurs beta cells to make more insulin	Easy to take; can be taken once a day; bothersome side effects are unusual; inexpensive	Wears out beta cells faster than other drugs; not proven to prevent blood vessel damage; can cause dangerously low blood sugar; promotes weight gain	The first kind of pills available for diabetes; falling out of favor because of lack of long-term benefit
Glipizide	Same as glyburide	Similar to glyburide; inexpensive	Same as glyburide	Raises after-meal insulin levels more than glyburide

14

Step 5
Making Up Any Insulin Deficit with Insulin

More so with diabetes than any other common, serious medical condition, how well you do is up to you. You need a doctor to get you started and give you advice on medications, but how successful you are at controlling it depends mainly on your actions—how closely you monitor your blood sugar, how carefully you avoid starch, how much attention you pay to exercise, and how willing you are to take medications if needed.

Moreover, it's openly acknowledged by medical organizations that when it comes to adult-onset diabetes, just consulting a doctor doesn't guarantee the best treatment. Doctors vary widely in how seriously they take type 2 diabetes. Some are satisfied just to keep their patients from experiencing bothersome symptoms caused by high blood sugar, such as frequent urination or dehydration. Indeed, most people with diabetes feel fine with fasting blood sugar levels between 150 and 200—low enough to avoid dehydration but nevertheless high enough to cause long-term complications such as damage to eyes, kidneys, and blood vessels.

The lower you try to get your blood sugar, the more medications you might have to take, which increases the risk of side effects. The most feared complication is hypoglycemia, low blood sugar. Excessive doses of some diabetes drugs can drive blood sugar levels low enough to cause mental confusion, coma, or even death. The specter of emergency room visits, car accidents, and lawsuits makes doctors and patients wary of pushing the blood sugar too low. It's easier—though not necessarily better for patients—to settle for less-than-ideal blood sugar levels.

Another reason many diabetics don't control their blood sugar levels well enough to prevent complications is a tendency for patients and doctors to want to treat things "naturally"—meaning without medication or with as little medication as possible. Indeed, many folks distrust pharmaceuticals. The media seem to jump at the opportunity to broadcast news of rare side effects of medications but rarely discuss the benefits.

There's also often an element of denial. It's hard to accept the fact that you have a disease that will require a lifetime of treatment, especially if you don't feel sick. For a while after I discovered I had diabetes, although I knew intellectually I would have it for life, I found myself hoping against hope that my case was some kind of an aberration—that my beta cells would somehow bounce back and I would be a whole person again. Of course, that didn't happen. It never does.

After a couple of months in which I watched my diet, exercised faithfully, and took metformin, my fasting blood sugar level had dropped from 380 to 150 or so—a lot better but still not normal. Like most patients, I would have liked to avoid taking insulin shots, but as a doctor, I had a different perspective. I had seen the damage that poorly controlled diabetes can do, and it was not a pretty picture. I knew that just keeping my blood sugar low enough to avoid symptoms was no guarantee against such complications.

In 1995, a few years before I discovered my diabetes, a large research trial called the United Kingdom Prospective Diabetes Study (UKPDS) reported that damage to eyes, kidneys, and blood vessels could be prevented if blood sugar levels were kept not just low enough to avoid dehydration but at near-normal levels. Those findings strengthened my resolve to keep my blood sugar levels as close to normal as possible. Indeed, the best results in that study were among patients who took the combination of metformin and insulin. I figured that if I wanted better control of my diabetes, the next step should be insulin.

Folks obviously dislike the idea of giving themselves shots. It's bad enough to have a nurse or doctor stick you with a needle during the occasional trip to the doctor, but the idea of injecting yourself every day can be hard to accept, especially if you feel OK to begin with. Of course, most of the hesitancy stems from fear of pain from the shots themselves. In addition, taking insulin seems more complicated than taking pills. You have to figure out how much insulin you need, which can vary with changes in your diet and physical activity. More worrisome, if you give yourself too much, you can push your blood sugar too low, which can be dangerous.

Although more convenient injection devices are available these days, when I first discovered my diabetes, you still had to draw insulin out of a vial with a needle and syringe each time you gave yourself a shot. That meant you had to learn to use sterile technique so you didn't contaminate the insulin. You also had to learn to keep yourself stocked with syringes, needles, alcohol swabs, and vials of insulin. Worst of all, you had to take this paraphernalia with you when you traveled or even went out to dinner.

Patients aren't the only ones who balk at the idea of treating type 2 diabetes with insulin. Sometimes physicians are reluctant, too. Nobody likes to be the bearer of bad news. Doctors understand that if patients are already watching their diet, exercising, and taking pills, the last thing they want to hear is that they should also give themselves insulin shots. Most people feel fine with fasting blood sugar levels between 150 and 200, so it's tempting for doctors to be reassuring about such readings. In addition, many doctors are unpracticed at teaching patients to use insulin. Often they have to refer patients to endocrinologists or diabetes educators to learn how to take insulin.

Make no mistake, if you are doing everything you're supposed to do—watching your diet, exercising regularly, and taking your liver-sensitizing pills—but your fasting blood sugar levels are still higher than normal, you are lacking in insulin, and that deficit is putting you at increased risk for eye, kidney, nerve, and blood vessel damage. Thankfully, modern technology has synthesized the exact insulin molecule your body makes. There is no better way to compensate for your beta cells' inability to make enough insulin than to supplement your body's own insulin with injected insulin.

Insulin rapidly removes glucose from your bloodstream. Insulin goes directly to the tissues of your body that need it, opens tiny gates in cell membranes, and lets glucose pass out of your bloodstream and into the cells where it belongs. In addition to helping you maintain normal blood sugar levels, injected insulin reduces the amount of insulin your beta cells have to make, which helps keep them from wearing out. By allowing your beta cells to conserve their own insulin, injected insulin makes it possible for those cells to contribute natural insulin when needed.

Healthy humans typically produce about thirty to forty units of natural insulin a day. In my experience, most type 2 diabetics who follow a low-starch diet, exercise regularly, and take insulin-sensitizing medication need less than thirty units a day of injected insulin to keep their fasting blood sugar levels near normal. Some only need ten to fifteen units.

People vary in their sensitivity to injected insulin. When you first start taking insulin, it's best to begin with a small dose to gauge its effect. I started by giving myself a small amount before dinner as a test dose, not expecting it to have much effect. The next morning, I was astonished to find that my blood sugar had gone down to 104, which is well below 125, the level at which doctors diagnose diabetes. I tried a little more the next night. The following morning it was 88. I did this several nights in a row, each time with similar results—perfectly normal fasting blood glucose levels.

That sold me. I didn't care if I had to poke myself with a needle every day for the rest of my life. The impressive effects insulin had on my blood sugar convinced me that insulin shots were the way to go—the magic bullet I had been looking for.

Looking back, I saw that cutting carbs, exercising, and taking insulin all made big differences in my getting from a fasting blood sugar of 380 to less than 100, while metformin had only a mild blood-sugar-lowering effect. I realized I probably could have controlled my blood sugar without metformin if I took more insulin. However, I knew that adult-onset diabetes is not just a disease of insulin deficiency but also of increased insulin needs. Insulin injections helped correct the insulin deficit, while metformin helped reduce my body's needs for insulin. Indeed, long-term results of the United Kingdom Prospective Diabetes Study have recently shown that metformin is even more effective at preventing complications than previously thought.

I procured a supply of insulin, disposable syringes, needles, and alcohol swabs. Every night before dinner—as I had taught many diabetics to do—I wiped off the top of an insulin vial with an alcohol swab, drew some air into a syringe, and injected it into the vial. I withdrew the amount of insulin I needed, wiped off a small area of skin on my thigh or belly with an alcohol swab, and injected the insulin about a third of an inch under my skin. I pressed on the spot with the swab for a few seconds to keep it from bleeding and then discarded the needle and syringe.

In a few weeks, I fell into a routine that worked great for keeping my blood sugar down. I had a light breakfast and a low-carb lunch, which was my usual pattern anyway. For dinner, I gave myself a shot of insulin, relaxed, and ate heartily.

Injecting myself away from home was indeed a nuisance. If I went to a restaurant or someone's house for dinner, I had to load my pockets with supplies first. To avoid *low* blood sugar, I had to wait until I was sure I was going to be served, then excuse myself—usually in the middle of a good conversation, it seemed— and find a bathroom where I could inject in private. Fumbling with a syringe in the shadowy recesses of a men's room never failed to elicit the feeling of being like a junkie shooting up in an alley.

You can skip shots. Nothing drastic happens. It would take several days for any symptoms from high blood sugar to develop if they indeed developed at all. Nevertheless, if you want consistently normal readings, you need to take your insulin as regularly as possible. There are times, of course, when you can't avoid being without insulin. I look upon these occasions as challenges in low-starch eating. If I meticulously avoid starch, my blood sugar levels are usually fine. If I have been taking my insulin regularly in the preceding days and am careful about what I eat, my beta cells seem to have enough insulin in reserve to handle the occasional missed dose.

As diabetics, we are indeed fortunate to live in this modern age of technology. It happened that a couple of months after I started taking insulin, a pharmaceutical representative came to my office to show me a new gadget that, in my opinion, is a revolutionary innovation in diabetes treatment. It's called an insulin pen. It looks like a writing pen but is actually an injecting device. It comes pre-loaded with 300 units of insulin—about a month's worth for me. It has a push-button on one end and a disposable needle on the other. To inject yourself, you just dial up the amount of insulin you need, poke yourself, and press the button. You can carry the device in your pocket like a pen. You no longer have to keep supplied with disposable syringes or draw insulin out of a vial every time you need a shot. I immediately abandoned my syringes and vials and went for the pen.

The insulin pen was especially liberating for me when I coupled it with another technique I had read about. Doctors and nurses are taught to use certain precautions when giving shots—baring the skin, wiping the skin with alcohol—the purpose being to avoid skin infections. However, nobody had actually studied these rituals systematically to see if they really were necessary. They just seemed like a good idea. Finally, some researchers put these rituals to the test. Reporting in the journal *Diabetes Care* in 1997, researchers at Wayne State University instructed fifty patients to omit the alcohol wipe and inject themselves right through their clothing. After twenty weeks and a total of 13,720 injections, there wasn't a single infection.

It makes sense to be as careful with injections as possible. I use the traditional technique when I'm giving myself shots at home. However, when I'm at a restaurant or someone's house for dinner, I often inject myself right through my clothing. I've found that I can take out my pen, hold it under the table and administer the shot through my pants without anyone noticing. I can actually carry on a conversation while I'm doing it. Not having to pack around vials, needles, or syringes or to leave the table to give myself shots makes it much easier to take insulin consistently.

In many ways, giving yourself insulin shots is easier than taking pills. Allergic reactions are rare. Gastrointestinal side effects are unheard of. You don't need to carry pills with you or find a glass of water to swallow them. If you need less than thirty units a day, it's cheaper than many diabetes pills.

I was also fortunate to be able to take advantage of some recent reformulations of insulin. Now you can choose from several kinds of insulin with different timing of action. Some are short-acting, exerting their effect quickly and clearing out of the bloodstream fast. Some are long-acting, creating a steady effect that lasts up to twenty-four hours. Others combine short- and long-acting preparations, giving a quick burst of strong action followed by a prolonged period of milder action. With different action profiles to choose from, you can duplicate your body's natural response to your particular eating and activity patterns.

I found I needed only a little insulin in my system to handle my daytime needs but a surge to handle my dinners. After trying various doses of different kinds of insulin, I have found that two shots—one shot of a mixture of short and intermediate-acting insulin and another shot of long-acting insulin—taken before dinner work well for me. Finding the right combination requires trying different doses, timing, and kinds of insulin. Indeed, it helped to be a doctor and have knowledge of the various preparations available and how they work. Tailoring insulin to your particular eating and exercise patterns involves a process of trial and error. The collaboration between doctor and patient needed to develop a good routine can be time-consuming. Unfortunately, the medical system often falls short in providing this important fine-tuning process. However, the right dose, timing, and kind of insulin can bring near-perfect control of blood sugar, and once you develop a routine that works, there's usually little need to change it for years at time.

Whereas small amounts of insulin actually suppress appetite and encourage weight loss, large amounts, whether produced by the body or taken as medication, can cause weight gain, which is the last thing you need if you have type 2 diabetes. Insulin is great medication even for mild diabetes. The trick is to take as much as you need to keep your blood sugar down but at the same time keeping your body's insulin requirements as low as possible.

Your need for insulin is like a three-legged stool. The legs are how much starch you eat, how sensitive your muscles are to insulin, and how much glucose your liver pours into your bloodstream. If you pay attention to all three of those factors, you can usually control your blood sugar with relatively small doses of insulin. If you neglect one of those legs, the stool will fall out of balance and you will need more insulin. Cutting out starch is of primary importance. In addition, you need to keep your muscles sensitive to insulin with exercise and prevent your liver from secreting glucose inappropriately with medication.

Before I started taking insulin, I felt like I was at the mercy of diabetes. All I could do was wonder what the disease was doing to me and wait for complications to develop. Insulin put me back in the driver's seat. My glucometer and pen did what my beta cells could not. I was in control of my life again. It has been ten years since I discovered my diabetes. Insulin, metformin, and the occasional "pasta pill" have been all the medication I have needed to keep my blood sugar levels normal. I have never had to increase the dosages.

The Folly of Not Taking Insulin When You Need It

Insulin treatment for diabetes has been one of the seminal advances of modern medicine. Perhaps because the medication has been around for seventy years, the excitement has worn off. Manufacturing patents have expired, and there are newer, more profitable drugs for pharmaceutical companies to sell. Nevertheless, insulin continues to save the lives of millions of patients with diabetes.

Because many patients with juvenile diabetes depend on insulin shots to survive, doctors sometimes refer to type 1 diabetes as "insulin-dependent" diabetes. Unfortunately, they then started calling type 2 diabetes "*non*-insulin-dependent" diabetes. This has led many patients and even some doctors to think that people with adult-onset diabetes don't need insulin unless their condition is far advanced. Being able to avoid insulin shots makes some patients think they're in good control of their diabetes or that they have a less serious form of the disease. Some doctors use the specter of insulin shots as a threat to get patients to lose weight, exercise, or take pills. It's not surprising that many patients regard insulin as the last resort, when it should be one of the first steps in treatment. It's certainly important to avoid starch and improve your body's sensitivity to insulin with exercise and insulin-sensitizing medication, but once those measures are in place, if your blood sugar is still high, you probably need to take insulin.

As for the fear of insulin injections, this is a groundless phobia, which usually disappears immediately when you give yourself the first shot. When patients try it, they usually feel silly about being so squeamish. It's a shame that many diabetics still suffer from irreversible vision loss, kidney failure, and heart disease because they are afraid to give themselves insulin shots. Needle phobia can be a deadly disease.

15

Step 6

Optimizing Your Cholesterol and Blood Pressure

I've always had a normal blood cholesterol level—normal before I developed diabetes, and normal afterward. However, according to national guidelines, I need to take cholesterol-lowering medication. Why would a person with a normal blood cholesterol level have to take medication to lower it further? Well, it turns out that if you have diabetes, "normal" isn't good enough. You need to keep your blood cholesterol level *lower than normal*. The same is true of your blood pressure. Here's why.

The Other Three Risk Factors for Blood Vessel Damage

Membranes surround every cell in your body and protect their inner environment. If your blood sugar level goes up, cell membranes regulate what goes in and out of cells and help keep potentially harmful substances from damaging them. However, your blood vessels are not similarly protected. They're directly exposed to whatever goes on in your blood, including high blood sugar, which is why the main complication of diabetes is blood vessel damage. But high blood sugar is not the only thing that can damage arteries. High blood levels of cholesterol—or more precisely, imbalances between good and bad cholesterol—also damage arteries, as do high concentrations of carbon monoxide from cigarette smoking. In addition, your arteries have to absorb the pressure that builds up in them as your heart pumps blood through them. High blood pressure also damages arteries.

Actually, blood vessels are really tough. In the absence of those four risk factors—high blood sugar, high blood pressure, cholesterol imbalances, and cigarette smoking—blood vessel problems are unusual. If you have mildly elevated blood sugar, as long as you don't have any of the other risk factors, your chances of developing blood vessel problems are not much higher than those of persons without diabetes. The problem is that diabetes sensitizes your blood vessels to the harmful effects of the other risk factors. In fact, for diabetics, having optimal blood pressure and cholesterol levels and stopping smoking are more important than having normal blood sugar levels.

"Normal" Versus "Ideal"

The four major risk factors for blood vessel disease—diabetes, high blood cholesterol, high blood pressure, and cigarette smoking—combine with one another to increase the risk of damage. The more of those risk factors you have and the more abnormal each is, the greater your risk. For example, if you have two risk factors, your risk is much higher than if you have just one. If you have three of those risk factors, your risk is higher than if you have two. Indeed, most people who have a heart attack or stroke have more than one of those risk factors.

Here's the key to preventing blood vessel damage and the reason I chose to take cholesterol-lowering medication even though my cholesterol level was normal. In the same way that risk factors can add to one another, *they can also subtract from one another.* Having a cholesterol level that is *lower* than normal can offset much of the risk of having a blood sugar level that is *higher* than normal. The same is true of blood pressure.

"Wait a minute," you might be thinking, "isn't it OK just to be normal?" In medicine, the word *normal* usually means "average," but average isn't necessarily best. For example, the average weight of Americans these days is higher than it should be for optimum health. This is also true for blood cholesterol levels and blood pressure. As far as your blood vessels are concerned, the lower your cholesterol and blood pressure, the better off you are, *even if they are below average.*

A word of caution: although there's no known downside to having a lower-than-average level of blood cholesterol, excessively low blood pressure can cause trouble. You need a certain amount of pressure in your arteries to push blood up to your head. If your blood pressure falls too low, it can cause dizziness or fainting.

Nevertheless, as far as the health of your blood vessels is concerned, ideal blood cholesterol and blood pressure levels are actually below-average levels. If you keep your blood pressure and cholesterol at ideal levels instead of just average levels, you can offset much of the risk of high blood sugar. Thanks to modern medicine, this is now easy to do.

Optimizing Your Blood Cholesterol Level

How well you control your blood *sugar* depends a lot on your lifestyle. It will fall dramatically if you cut out starch and exercise regularly. Your blood *cholesterol* level is another matter. Contrary to popular conception, the levels of bad blood cholesterol in your blood don't change much with lifestyle changes. High blood cholesterol is *not* caused by eating cholesterol-containing foods. Your body makes its own cholesterol—about three times more than you eat. If you eat less, it just makes more, and vice versa. Moreover, most of the cholesterol you eat passes right through your intestinal tract and out in your stool. The level of cholesterol in your blood is not a matter of how much cholesterol goes into your body; it's a matter of how much your body chooses to let out, and that's a genetic characteristic. Everybody's system has a genetically determined "set point" for eliminating cholesterol.

You might be thinking that if people's cholesterol levels are genetically determined, a lot of people must have genetic defects.

That's indeed true; the human gene pool is full of genetic defects of cholesterol metabolism, but doctors don't call them defects. They refer to them as "polymorphisms." We'll just call them "quirks."

You might wonder why Mother Nature allowed humans to have so many genetic quirks in their cholesterol metabolism. Well, in prehistoric times, it didn't matter what your cholesterol level was. Humans didn't live long enough for high blood cholesterol to cause trouble. Most humans died before age thirty. Minor genetic quirks of cholesterol metabolism accumulated harmlessly in the gene pool for millions of years. Only since humans started living longer have these defects significantly influenced health and longevity.

Since genes rather than diet determine your cholesterol level, it's not surprising that low-cholesterol diets don't work very well for lowering blood cholesterol levels. As discussed in Chapter 4, strict low-fat, low-cholesterol diets supervised by professional dietitians reduce levels of bad cholesterol at best between 5 and 10 percent, which doesn't put much of a dent in your risk of blood vessel problems. To put that in perspective, modern cholesterol-lowering drugs can lower bad cholesterol by as much as 60 percent and raise good cholesterol, which significantly reduces the risk.

If you have diabetes or insulin resistance, there is, in fact, some serious downsides to trying to cut out fat and cholesterol. Namely, you have to eat something, so you usually end up eating more starch, which, because of your diabetes, is much more harmful than dietary cholesterol. Not only does increasing starch consumption raise blood sugar, it also increases triglyceride levels and lowers the level of good cholesterol in your blood, which makes it easier for harmful cholesterol particles to build up in your blood vessels and cause damage. Low-fat diets actually reduce levels of good cholesterol and often worsen the balance between good and bad cholesterol.

What about exercise? It's great for lowering blood sugar. In fact, you can't control diabetes very well without it. It also lowers the triglyceride in your blood and raises good-cholesterol levels, which is important. However, studies have repeatedly shown that exercise does not reduce blood levels of bad cholesterol.

If diet and exercise don't reduce bad cholesterol enough to do you much good, what *can* you do about high blood cholesterol? Liver cells have tiny receptors on their surfaces that pluck cholesterol particles out of the bloodstream and allow it to break those particles down and eliminate them. The reason some people's bodies don't get rid of cholesterol as readily as others' do is that their cholesterol receptors are genetically less active.

In the 1980s, two American scientists won the Nobel Prize for deciphering the enzyme systems that control the amount of cholesterol receptors on liver cells. Soon pharmaceutical companies developed medications that could switch on those enzyme systems so they would put more cholesterol receptors on the liver cells. The medications, called statins, correct the genetic quirks that cause high blood cholesterol. Doctors now have highly effective cholesterol-lowering medication, including lovastatin (trade name Mevacor), pravastatin (Pravachol), simvastatin (Zocor), fluvastatin (Lescol), atorvatstatin (Lipitor), and rosuvastatin (Crestor). One pill a day is usually all that's needed to reduce blood cholesterol levels not just to normal, but to ideal levels.

How Low Is Ideal?

When making decisions about treating high cholesterol, doctors don't just look at the total concentration of cholesterol in your blood. They look at the levels of bad cholesterol, called LDL, and good cholesterol, or HDL. The average LDL level of Americans is approximately 140. For people who don't have diabetes or other risk factors for blood vessel disease, the National Institutes of Health guidelines for treating cholesterol recommend keeping the LDL level less than 160. However, for people with diabetes, even if they have no other risk factors for blood vessel disease, the guidelines recommend keeping the LDL level less than 100. That means that most people with adult-onset diabetes, even if their LDL is below average, should take cholesterol-lowering medication.

Here's some good news: if you take a statin, you can usually eat all the fat and cholesterol you want (within reason) without raising your cholesterol. Statins allow any excess cholesterol to pass right out of your system. Indeed, if you have diabetes or pre-diabetes, you are better off focusing on eliminating starch instead of worrying about cholesterol. Not only does reducing starch make diabetes easier to control, it lowers triglyceride levels, raises HDL, and helps prevent the remaining LDL particles in the blood from infiltrating and damaging blood vessels.

Side effects of statins are unusual. The most common is muscle soreness, which affects about one in twenty people who take them. This can often be relieved by lowering the dosage and adding a different kind of cholesterol-lowering medication to rev up the cholesterol-lowering effects of the reduced statin.

Dangerous side effects are rare. The main one is muscle damage, which can occasionally be severe enough to injure the kidneys. If you have severe muscle soreness or weakness, you should stop the medication and call your doctor.

Optimizing Your Blood Pressure

High blood pressure also increases the damage that diabetes does to blood vessels. The pressure in your arteries rises and falls with each beat of your heart. The peak to which it rises with each beat is called the *systolic* pressure; the depth to which it falls is the *diastolic* pressure. Normal blood pressure for healthy young adults is less than 120 systolic and 80 diastolic, expressed as 120/80. The higher your blood pressure, the higher your risk of blood vessel disease. For people who do not have diabetes, the National Institutes of Health recommends treatment for blood pressure levels higher than 140/90.

Because diabetes makes blood vessels vulnerable to the harmful effects of high blood pressure, you can reduce your risk of blood vessel damage by making sure you treat high blood pressure. You can reduce your risk even further if you keep your blood pressure not just at levels usually considered normal, but at lower-than-normal levels. The American College of Cardiology guidelines recommend that people with diabetes try to keep their blood pressure lower than 130/85.

One problem with treating high blood pressure is figuring out what your true blood pressure is. Blood pressure varies from day to day, hour to hour, and even moment to moment. If it's way over the limit every time you measure it, you can reasonably conclude that it's high enough to require treatment. However, it might be high sometimes and fine at other times. Even people with ideal blood pressure levels sometimes have high readings when they're nervous or excited.

When your doctor checks your blood pressure, you should be relaxed, sitting calmly, and not talking. If the first reading is high, the doctor should immediately repeat it twice and base judgments on the lowest of the three readings. If there's a question as to whether your blood pressure is high or not, you should measure it again after a month or so.

As you age, your arteries naturally stiffen, which raises your systolic blood pressure. Indeed, if you live long enough, eventually your systolic pressure will probably exceed 140, the point at which the national guidelines usually recommend treatment. Systolic pressures higher than 140 are quite common in people older than fifty. However, "common" does not mean harmless. High blood pressure still puts pressure on arteries, and treatment to lower it helps prevent blood vessel damage.

Reducing systolic pressure when the diastolic pressure is already normal can be tricky. For one thing, systolic blood pressure varies a lot, and it's often difficult to tell how high it usually is. In addition, blood pressure medication can cause the blood pressure to fall too low, which can be dangerous.

Keeping your blood pressure at optimal levels is often as easy as taking one pill a day, especially if you start treatment early, when your blood pressure is just starting to rise above desirable levels. However, sometimes lowering it to the desirable range requires two or three different pills.

Considering that you're already taking medication for your diabetes and probably for your cholesterol, you probably aren't enthusiastic about taking more pills. If that's how you're feeling, take a deep breath. Be grateful that type 2 diabetes need not keep you from living to a ripe old age. It's just that you thought diabetes was a one-number disease when it's really a *three*-number disease—blood sugar, blood cholesterol, and blood pressure. The good news is that if you get those three numbers where they need to be, you can relax. Your diabetes will have gone from being a tiger to a pussycat. It will be in perfect control.

Part 3

Low-Starch Cuisine: Discovering a Tastier Way to Eat

Because starch is essentially a tasteless paste, if you replace it with other foods, you end up increasing the amount of flavor and texture in your diet. Indeed, eliminating starch can broaden your palate. Don't be surprised if you find yourself eating better than you did before you discovered your diabetes.

It's easy to find good low-starch recipes; unless a recipe is specifically for a baked good or a potato or rice dish, it's unlikely to contain much starch. I included some favorites in my book *The Glycemic-Load Diet*. Dana Carpender, one of America's most popular authors of low-carb cookbooks, provides 150 low-starch recipes in her book *The Glycemic-Load Diet Cookbook*.

American dietary tradition, born of economic necessity, dictates that we have a starch—bland, repetitive, and unexciting as it might be—with most meals. We're accustomed to having bread, potatoes, or rice on the table and intermingling their bland and pasty consistencies with other foods. If you miss those mealtime starches, take heart. With a little ingenuity you can create some delicious starch substitutes that not only look like and have consistency similar to bread, potatoes, and rice but actually taste better than those tired old starches. In Chapter 16, Dana will tell you how to make some of her favorite starch substitutes, which you will probably find are more delicious than the actual starches. (Don't pass up her delicious potato stand-in, Faux-tatoes.)

Most baked goods are made with wheat flour, which is pure starch. In fact, wheat is where Americans get most of their starch. As it turns out, there are several other kinds of flour that are just as good as wheat flour and won't raise your blood sugar. These might be a little more expensive than wheat flour, and you need to learn a few tricks to use them. However, with a little attention to detail, you can use these flours to prepare baked goods that are every bit as satisfying as the baked goods you're used to. I asked Dana to give us a lesson on using nonstarch flours to prepare baked goods and provide us with a few low-starch, baked-good recipes, which you will find in Chapter 17. Chapter 18 describes a seven-day low-glycemic-load meal plan. It will show you that eliminating starch opens the door not just to a healthier eating style but also to a tastier one.

16

Starch Substitutes That Taste Better than Starch

by Dana Carpender

Successful change requires strategy. It's about how you shop, what you keep in your kitchen, and what restaurants you choose. If you keep on stocking all your favorite starchy foods, you'll fall flat on your face in no time. If you're living on processed, frozen, and microwavable stuff and cooking as little as possible, you'll inevitably end up eating starch—and lots of it.

Accept that your low-starch diet is not going to look exactly like your old diet. It's just not. Try new recipes. Change food traditions. The more things you try, the more likely you are to hit on new favorites. And remember, "different" does not mean "worse."

Go to your local library and look through the cookbooks —particularly for new and interesting things to do with non-starchy vegetables. Moving beyond plain buttered vegetables and simple salads will give new life to your menus. Look, too, for low-carbohydrate diet cookbooks, since low-carbohydrate recipes are usually low-starch recipes.

Look, you have to do this for the rest of your life to keep from going blind and losing your toes. So get in the game!

Breads

Bread, rolls, buns, tortillas, pita—starch bombs, every one, yet we have been programmed to eat them at every meal. Americans have become sandwich junkies. We eat on the run and want food we can eat while we drive. This does not make for good nutrition *or* safe driving! And really, all the bread does is act as an edible napkin.

Let me introduce you to a miraculous invention: the fork. This astonishing, high-tech tool lets you pick up foods and put them in your mouth without dirtying your hands, without the use of bread. *Wow!* It's hard to operate this technology while driving a car, but that's just a sacrifice you're going to have to make. Take a big five minutes to eat something decent, and save years of trouble down the road.

You can eat tuna, egg, ham, turkey, and chicken salads with a fork, wrap them in lettuce, or stuff them in celery. The fillings of most sandwiches make great main-dish salads—imagine all of the cold cuts of a traditional Italian hero on a big bed of crisp lettuce, with Italian vinaigrette dressing. Yum! The insides of gyros—meat, tsatsiki sauce, and all—piled on a Greek salad, with lots of feta and olives, is food for the Greek gods. Barbecued pulled pork on a big pile of crisp, creamy cole slaw? I'm making myself hungry!

Also, most sandwich fillings make great omelets. Consider the following combinations:

- Ham and cheddar, with a little mustard
- Leftover tuna salad with Swiss
- Turkey and provolone with a little mayo
- Monterey Jack and avocado slices with alfalfa sprouts

- Roast beef, sliced tomatoes, and horseradish
- Turkey, bacon, and sliced tomatoes

About the only sandwich filling I can think of that doesn't work as a salad or an omelet is peanut butter and jelly!

There are a few low-carb—and therefore low-starch—breads available. Read labels in the bread aisle at your grocery store, especially breads labeled "light" or "diet." Look at the numbers for total carbohydrate and fiber, and subtract the fiber from the carbohydrate. If the difference is five grams or lower, you can afford to eat that bread *in moderation*—a few slices a week, *not* a sandwich every day.

Low-carb tortillas also are available. Again, subtract the fiber content from the total carbohydrate content, and look for less than five grams of nonfiber carbohydrate per tortilla. I like La Tortilla Factory brand, each with twelve grams of carbohydrate—nine grams of which is fiber! That leaves just three grams of starchy carbohydrate per tortilla. (They also have a large size, which has nineteen grams of carb, of which fourteen grams are fiber, for just five grams of starchy carbohydrate per tortilla.) If you must have sandwiches, low-carb tortilla wraps are your best choice. If you can't find low-carb tortillas locally, shop online.

Do *not* mistake whole-grain bread or tortillas for low-carbohydrate or low-starch ones. Most whole-grain products have *more* starch per piece than white, not less. You must subtract the fiber from the total carbohydrate count to find the number of starchy-carb grams in bread and tortillas.

A few low-starch crackers are on the market. Wasa Fiber Rye, Finn Crisp, Bran-a-crisp, and FiberRich crackers all are low enough in starch and high enough in fiber that they can fit into your program in moderation.

Potato and Rice Substitutes

You know the stuff that fills up a third of your plate? You need to come up with something to take up that space! The single most useful substitute for starchy side dishes, believe it or not, is cauliflower. If you've only experienced cauliflower that is overcooked and topped with Cheez Whiz, you may be doubting, but please bear with me.

Here are two foundational recipes that will allow you to create dozens, if not hundreds, of side dishes, and I'll give you an example or two of how to use each one.

Faux-tatoes

Do try these, especially if you're making a good sauce or gravy. I can't tell you how many times I've had guests shovel in three or four forkfuls of Faux-tatoes and gravy before they say, "Wait a minute. That's not mashed potatoes. What—what is it?" No one has ever guessed it was cauliflower!

½ large cauliflower head

Trim the bottom of the stem, and remove leaves. Whack the rest into chunks, and throw 'em in a microwavable casserole with a lid. Add a couple of tablespoons of water, cover, and nuke on high for 12 to 14 minutes, until tender.

When your cauliflower is soft, drain it well. Use a regular blender, stick blender, or food processor to puree it. I use a stick blender and puree it right in the serving bowl.

Add butter, salt, pepper, and whatever you might add to mashed potatoes. An ounce or so of cream cheese melted in is fantastic.

Vary this recipe in any way you would mashed potatoes. Add shredded cheese, a clove of garlic, snipped herbs, pesto, sour cream and chives, a little barbecue sauce, or whatever will complement your main dish.

Nutrient information: 3 servings, each with 24 calories, trace fat, 2 g protein, 5 g carbohydrate, 2 g dietary fiber (This is the count for the cauliflower alone. Butter, cream cheese, or anything else you add will, of course, change the counts.)

Note: For a texture and flavor even closer to mashed potatoes, try cutting up just 6 ounces of potato and steaming it with the cauliflower, and then mash the two together. The nutrient information for 3 servings will be 69 calories, trace fat, 3 g protein, 15 g carbohydrate, 3 g dietary fiber.

Sour Cream Faux-tato Casserole

Here's a terrific faux-tato casserole that will dress up any plain main dish.

> 1 large cauliflower head
> 4 scallions
> 1 cup sour cream
> 2 tablespoons butter
> ¾ cup grated Parmesan cheese, divided
> Salt and pepper
> 1 teaspoon onion powder
> 1 teaspoon salt or Vege-Sal
> Paprika

Preheat oven to 350°F. Spray an 8-inch square baking pan with nonstick cooking spray.

Trim the bottom of the stem of your cauliflower, and remove the leaves. Whack the rest into big chunks, put it in a microwavable casserole with a lid or a microwave steamer if you have one, and add a few tablespoons of water. Cover and microwave on high for 15 to 18 minutes, or until quite tender.

While the cauliflower is cooking, slice your scallions thin, including the crisp part of the green shoot.

When your cauliflower is soft, drain it very well. Using your regular blender, stick blender, or food processor, puree the cauliflower along with the sour cream, butter, ½ cup Parmesan, onion powder, and salt or Vege-Sal and pepper to taste. Stir in the scallions by hand, and spread the mixture in your prepared baking dish. Sprinkle the remaining ¼ cup Parmesan on top, and dust lightly with paprika.

Bake for 40 to 45 minutes, and serve hot.

Nutrient information: 6 servings, each with 166 calories, 15 g fat, 6 g protein, 3 g carbohydrate, trace dietary fiber

Unpotato and Leek Soup

Here's another way pureed cauliflower can stand in for mashed potatoes. This thick and hearty soup is wonderful on a cold, sleety night.

　　3 leeks
　　2 celery ribs
　　4 tablespoons butter, divided
　　1 large head cauliflower
　　2 quarts chicken stock
　　2 bay leaves
　　1 clove garlic, crushed
　　1½ teaspoons dried thyme
　　¼ teaspoon ground allspice
　　½ teaspoon dried mustard powder
　　1 pound smoked sausage
　　1 teaspoon guar or xanthan
　　2 cups half-and-half

Trim the greens off the leeks just above the compact, cylindrical part. Slice each leek vertically up the middle from the root to the top, leaving the roots intact on each half. Fan out your cut leeks under running water, and wash between the layers—leeks can hold a lot of grit.

Slice your leeks thinly into half-rounds. Dice your celery, including any leaves.

In a big stock pot, over medium heat, melt 3 tablespoons of the butter, and throw in the leeks and celery. Sauté, stirring often, until they're soft. Don't let them brown. Meanwhile, chop up your cauliflower into 1-inch chunks.

When the leeks and celery are soft, throw in the cauliflower, chicken stock, bay leaves, garlic, thyme, allspice, and mustard powder. Bring to a simmer, and let it cook for a good 45 minutes to an hour, until the cauliflower is soft.

While the soup is simmering, slice your smoked sausage lengthwise and then across into bite-sized pieces. Sauté them in the remaining tablespoon of butter till brown on both sides, and then just turn off the burner and let 'em wait in the skillet.

When the cauliflower is tender, you need to puree your soup. The easiest way is with a stick blender, right in the pot, or use a slotted spoon to transfer the vegetables into your regular blender or food processor. However you puree the veggies, add the teaspoon of guar or xanthan while you're doing it. If you've used a regular blender or food processor, dump your puree back into your stock pot.

Now stir in those sausage slices! Use a ladleful of your soup to rinse all the brown, flavorful stuff out of the skillet, and pour that into the soup, too.

Stir in the half-and-half, let the whole thing simmer another 10 minutes, and serve.

Nutrient information: 6 servings, each with 512 calories, 41 g fat, 16 g protein, 18 g carbohydrate, 4 g dietary fiber

Unpotato Salad

I have made at least a dozen different potato salad recipes with cauliflower in place of potatoes, and all of them have worked out brilliantly.

Simply cut your cauliflower into ½-inch chunks, and steam it for about 8 to 10 minutes, or until tender but not mushy. Use just like potatoes in any potato salad recipe. Wonderful!

Scalloped Turnips

Another good stand-in for potatoes is turnips. While ½ cup of potatoes has 12 grams of starch, ½ cup of turnips has only 3 grams. I like them in stews and soups; when they've been simmered for a long time in a flavorful broth or gravy, it's hard to tell the difference. Try them in vegetable-beef soup or your favorite beef stew recipe. Turnips are also great pan-roasted with lamb or roast beef, scalloped, or au gratin.

This recipe makes a great side dish with a roast. We had it with our ham for Christmas dinner, and it was wonderful.

> 5 medium turnips
> 2 tablespoons butter
> 1 medium onion, diced fine
> 2 cloves garlic, crushed
> 1½ teaspoons dried thyme, or 1 tablespoon fresh thyme leaves
> 1¼ teaspoons salt, or to taste
> ¼ teaspoon pepper
> 1 cup chicken broth, or 1 cup water plus 1 teaspoon chicken bouillon concentrate
> 1 cup heavy cream
> 2 whole bay leaves
> 8 ounces cheddar cheese, shredded
> ½ cup grated Parmesan cheese
> Guar or xanthan

Peel your turnips, and run them through the slicing blade of your food processor. (If you don't have a food processor, slice 'em about ⅛ inch thick.) Set them aside.

Melt the butter in a Dutch oven over medium heat. Add the onion and sauté till it's getting golden and translucent. Now add the garlic, thyme, salt, and pepper, and sauté together for another minute or two.

Now add the sliced turnips, chicken broth, cream, and bay leaves. Turn the heat down, cover the Dutch oven, and let the whole thing simmer for a good half hour, till the turnips are nearly tender.

In the meantime, preheat your oven to 375°F, and coat an 8-inch square baking dish with nonstick cooking spray.

When the turnips are al dente, scoop half of 'em out with a slotted spoon, and transfer them into the prepared baking dish. Scatter half of the cheeses over them. Scoop out the rest of the turnips and make a second layer. (Somewhere in this process you will run across those bay leaves. Pull 'em out and discard 'em.)

Now wait a second before adding the rest of the cheese! Use your guar or xanthan shaker and a whisk to thicken up the cream/broth mixture in the Dutch oven to the consistency of heavy cream. Ladle it over the turnips in the baking dish.

Top with the rest of the cheese. Slide it into the oven, and let it bake till the cheese is just turning brown—45 minutes or so. Serve hot!

Nutrient information: 8 servings, each with 298 calories, 25 g fat, 11 g protein, 8 g carbohydrate, 2 g dietary fiber

Cauli-Rice

Now a replacement for rice: Fran McCullough, a far better cook-book writer than I, invented this, and I've been running with it ever since. I've used Cauli-Rice in everything from "rice" or "couscous" salads to pilafs to fried "rice" to jambalaya.

½ large cauliflower head

Trim the bottom of the stem, and cut off the leaves. Whack the rest of your cauliflower into chunks, and run it through the shredding blade of your food processor.

Put the resulting "rice" in a microwavable casserole with a lid, add a couple of tablespoons of water, cover, and nuke on high for 6 minutes. Uncover promptly when the microwave beeps, to stop cooking and prevent mushiness.

Nutrient information: 3–4 servings; assuming 3, each has 18 calories, trace fat, 1 g protein, 4 g carbohydrate, 2 g dietary fiber

Savory "Rice"

Rice is often cooked in broth, but of course cauliflower won't absorb all that liquid. Instead, season Cauli-Rice with bouillon concentrate. (I like Better Than Bouillon meat bases, but granules or liquid will do. Cubes are hard to use here.) Use whatever flavor goes with your main course—beef bouillon with beef, chicken bouillon with chicken, etc. Add sautéed onions or sliced scallions, herbs to complement the meal, maybe some chopped nuts or sautéed mushrooms—the options are limitless.

I adapted this from a recipe in a soul food cookbook. It was great with braised pork chops and gravy!

½ large cauliflower head
3 tablespoons butter
1 medium onion, chopped
1½ teaspoons dried thyme
2 teaspoons chicken bouillon granules
Salt and pepper

Trim the bottom of your cauliflower stem, and cut off the leaves. Whack the rest into chunks, and run it through the shredding blade of your food processor. Put the resulting "rice" in a microwavable casserole with a lid, add a couple of tablespoons of water, cover, and nuke on high for 6 minutes.

While that's cooking, melt the butter in your big, heavy skillet over medium heat, and throw in the chopped onion. Sauté till soft and turning golden.

Right about now, the microwave should beep. Drain the cooked Cauli-Rice and add it to the skillet. Add the thyme and bouillon concentrate, and stir till everything is very well combined and evenly distributed.

Salt and pepper to taste, stir again, and serve.

Nutrient information: 4 servings, each with 109 calories, 9 g fat, 2 g protein, 7 g carbohydrate, 2 g dietary fiber

Maggie's Crustless Mini Quiches

Quiche is a delicacy you don't want to live without. It usually has a starchy crust, like a pie, but the tasty part, the filling, is actually starch free. You can push the crust aside if you want, but why even bother preparing the crust? You can cook up a batch of these muffin-pan quiches, which are small enough to maintain their form without a crust. You can eat some right away, or you can stick some in your freezer and microwave them for a quick meal later.

> 1 tablespoon butter
> ¼ cup diced yellow onion
> ¼ cup diced green pepper
> ¼ cup cubed ham
> 6 eggs
> ¼ cup cream or milk
> ¼ cup shredded cheddar cheese

Preheat oven to 375°F. Line a muffin pan with foil cupcake wrappers (paper ones will not work). If you choose not to use wrappers, grease the tin thoroughly.

In a skillet, melt the butter over medium-high heat. Add the onions, then the peppers, and sauté. Add salt and pepper to taste. Mix in the cubed ham, and remove from heat.

Next, break the eggs into a large measuring cup with a pouring spout or a bowl. Beat the eggs, and add the cream.

Scoop a spoonful of the pepper, onion, and ham mixture into the bottom of each muffin cup. Sprinkle with a pinch of shredded cheese. Pour or ladle the egg mixture into the cups, covering the other ingredients. Cups should be about ½ to ⅔ full. Do not fill them all the way, because the mixture expands when cooked.

Bake for 20 to 25 minutes, or until golden brown on top. Remove finished quiches from oven, and allow them to cool for at least 5 minutes before attempting to remove them from the tin, especially if you did not use liners. Gently run a knife around the edges of the cups to loosen them from the tin. Flip the tin upside down over a plate and give it a few pats to remove the quiches.

You can substitute any of your favorite omelet ingredients and cheeses for the quiche fillings. All vegetables should be sautéed first to cook out the excess water.

Nutrient information: 6 servings, each with 117 calories, 8 g fat, 9 g protein, 2 g carbohydrate, 0.2 g dietary fiber

Noodles, Macaroni, Spaghetti, and Other Pasta

I know there are many noodle lovers. If you're among them, I'm afraid you'll have to reform. Most pasta, even whole wheat pasta, is loaded with starch. There are a few substitutes to consider.

Dreamfields pasta has a taste and texture identical to regular pasta, because the ingredients are very similar, though with more fiber. But Dreamfields claims it has a special process that keeps you from digesting and absorbing much of the starch in its pasta, yielding only five grams per serving. I have doubts. I have tested my blood sugar after eating Dreamfields on an empty stomach, and my blood sugar jumped more than it should have from just five grams of starch, though less than it would from regular pasta. Nevertheless, I have heard from diabetic readers who find that it does not mess up their blood sugar—and even from people who say it sometimes messes up their blood sugar and other times does not.

So try Dreamfields if you like, but be cautious. Eat it in modest quantities, along with plenty of protein and low-starch vegetables. And keep a close eye on your blood sugar; if it jumps after you eat Dreamfields, you know the stuff is not for you.

Spaghetti Squash

Spaghetti squash works well in a lot of recipes. I've used it in casserole recipes—even my grandma's best casserole!—with great success. I've also made spaghetti squash carbonara, Alfredo, pad thai—you name it.

1 spaghetti squash

To cook a spaghetti squash, stab it all over with a fork, and then throw it in the microwave on high for 12 to 14 minutes. When it's cool enough to handle, split it in half, scoop out the seeds, and then scrape the flesh with a fork. It will separate into spaghetti-like strands, which is quite amazing the first time you do it. Use it in all manner of recipes.

Nutrient information: 1 cup of cooked spaghetti squash has just 7 g carbohydrate (compared with 40 g in a cup of cooked spaghetti!), 31 calories, 1 g fat, 7 g carb, 0 g fiber, 1 g protein

Nadine's Zucchini Lasagna

Dr. Rob's nurse, Nadine, has been serving her family this delicious lasagna made with flat slices of zucchini instead of pasta for years, not because of its low starch content but because it tastes so good.

> 4 medium (10-ounce) zucchini squash
> 2 cups ricotta cheese
> 3 eggs
> 1 pound hamburger
> 4 cups (2 medium size cans) tomato sauce
> 2 tablespoons Italian seasoning or oregano
> 1 teaspoon salt and pepper
> 1 tablespoon butter
> ½ cup grated Parmesan cheese

Cut the zucchini lengthwise into flat ¼-inch slices. In a bowl, blend the ricotta with the eggs using a hand mixer. Brown the hamburger in a saucepan and then add to the tomato sauce and ricotta, add seasoning, and stir. Coat a baking dish (approximately 13 by 19 inches) with butter, put a third of the mixture on the bottom, cover with a layer of zucchini, and repeat twice so that you have three layers of sauce alternating with zucchini. Bake at 350° F for 45 minutes. Remove from oven, sprinkle Parmesan on top and bake for 7 more minutes to melt cheese.

Nutrient information: 8 servings, each with 366 calories, 23 g fat, 26 g protein, 15 g carbohydrate, 0.5 g dietary fiber

Shirataki Noodles

There is a truly starch-free noodle available; it is also very low in calories. It's a traditional Japanese noodle called *shirataki*. These noodles are made from fiber and virtually nothing else! There are two types, traditional shirataki and tofu shirataki. The traditional version is clear and sort of gelatinous; it's best in Asian dishes like sesame noodles or pad thai. Tofu shirataki is white and has a texture that is more similar to the noodles we're used to. Tofu shirataki noodles come in spaghetti-like strands and fettuccine-like strips. The fettuccine-style tofu shirataki noodles work well in all sorts of dishes. They're good with tomato sauce and Parmesan, make a great fettuccine Alfredo, and even are good in tuna-noodle casserole.

Shirataki noodles come already hydrated—you don't have to boil them—in plastic pouches full of liquid. You snip open the pouch, dump them into a strainer, and rinse them. You'll notice that the liquid smells fishy; don't worry about it. I've never noticed a fish taste in my finished dishes.

Find shirataki noodles in Asian markets and many health food stores, or order them online. Unopened, they will keep for months in your fridge, so feel free to stock up.

Here are a couple of ways I've used shirataki recently.

Chicken Lo Mein

Confession: The day I invented this, I ate half of it for lunch. It was so good, I went back and ate the rest. Then I could barely move for the rest of the day!

Do all your preparation before you start cooking.

> 1 package shirataki noodles—tofu, fettucine style
> 10 ounces chicken breast, no skin, no bone, RTC
> 1 cup Chinese cabbage, sliced
> ½ cup sliced celery
> 4 scallions, cut ½ inch long, including the crisp part of the green shoot
> 1 cup mung bean sprouts
> 2 tablespoons soy sauce
> 1 tablespoon dry sherry
> 1 tablespoon grated gingerroot
> 1 clove garlic, crushed
> ¼ teaspoon Splenda or sugar
> 2 tablespoons peanut oil or coconut oil

Snip open your packet of shirataki noodles, and dump them into a strainer (over the sink, of course!). Rinse well. Use your kitchen shears to snip across them in a few different directions, because in their natural state, they're too darned long.

Cut your chicken breast into ½-inch cubes. Put 'em on a plate next to the stove.

Slice your Chinese cabbage, across the whole head, about ¼ inch thick. Thin-slice your celery. Cut your scallions into ½-inch lengths. Measure the bean sprouts. Put all these vegetables on another plate, and set it by the stove, too.

In a small dish, combine the soy sauce, sherry, gingerroot, garlic, and Splenda. Stir it up. Set this by the stove as well.

OK, you're ready to cook! Put your wok or a big skillet over highest heat. When it's good and hot, add the oil, and throw in the chicken. Stir-fry it until all the pink is gone. Scoop it out of the wok, and transfer it back onto the plate. (Yes, I know the plate has raw-chicken germs on it. You're going to heat the chicken again, so don't panic.)

If you need a little more oil, add it, and dump in the vegetables. Stir-fry for just a minute or two—all of these vegetables cook very quickly.

When the veggies are just tender-crisp, throw the chicken back in the wok, and add the soy sauce mixture. Stir it all up. Turn the burner down to medium-low.

Stir in the shirataki noodles, and let the whole thing simmer for just a minute or two more, then serve.

Nutrient information: 2 servings, each with 364 calories, 18 g fat, 36 g protein, 13 g carbohydrate, 5 g dietary fiber

Grandma's Chicken Noodle Soup

The ultimate comfort food! Easy, too. The flavor of this soup depends on the quality of your broth. It's worth trying several brands to see which you like best.

> 1 quart chicken broth
> 1 carrot, peeled and sliced
> 1 celery rib, diced
> 8 ounces boneless, skinless chicken breast or thigh (see recipe note)
> 1 8-ounce package fettuccine-style tofu shirataki noodles
> Salt and pepper

Notice, please, the nice, simple quantities in the ingredients list. If ever a recipe was made for easy multiplying, this is it.

Put the broth in a kettle or slow cooker. Cut up the carrot and celery, and throw them in. Bring it to a simmer, or cover your slow cooker and set to low or high, depending on how much time you have (if you have all day, low; if you've got only a few hours, high). However you heat your broth and veggies, let the whole thing simmer till the carrot and celery are soft. (On the stove, this will take 30 to 45 minutes.)

Cut your chicken into ½-inch cubes, and stir it into the hot soup. (Don't just dump it in and let it sit, or it will congeal into a big lump at the bottom of the pot.) If you're using a slow cooker and it has been on low, turn it up to high. Otherwise, just let your soup keep simmering. Give it another 20 to 30 minutes.

While the chicken is simmering, cut open your shirataki packet, and dump the noodles into a strainer. Rinse 'em, and then snip across them a few times with your kitchen shears. Now dump 'em into your soup.

Add salt and pepper to taste, and you're done! Serve 'er up.

Nutrient information: 4 servings, each with 125 calories, 3 g fat, 18 g protein, 5 g carbohydrate, 2 g dietary fiber

Note: Cubing the chicken is easiest if it's half-frozen.

Macaroni and Cheese

Try tofu fettuccine-style shirataki in your favorite mac-and-cheese recipe. If you buy cheddar cheese powder (mentioned in the Chee-Fauxs recipe—see Index), you can use it just like the cheese packet in the good ol' standard boxed macaroni and cheese. I use one packet of tofu shirataki fettucini, the cheese packet from a package of mac and cheese, ¼ cup butter, and ¼ cup milk. This makes a fair amount of sauce for that many noodles, so you could probably increase it to a packet and a half or two packets of noodles. If you're using cheddar powder, start with a couple of tablespoons and then increase if you wish.

Breakfast Cereal

Even supposedly "healthy" stuff like granola, oatmeal, and whole-grain cold cereals are wildly starchy and will jack your blood sugar around but good. The only cereals in your grocery store that are OK—not great, but OK—are the spaghetti-shaped bran cereals, All-Bran (and especially All-Bran Extra Fiber) and Fiber One. If you want a small serving of one of these for breakfast, OK, but have some protein, too.

My favorite way to eat these cereals is to throw a few sliced strawberries in a bowl, add Splenda-sweetened vanilla yogurt, and top with a handful of bran cereal, for crunch. This makes a great summer breakfast.

Check the low-carb online stores for low-carb (and therefore low-starch) granolas.

Snacks

You know that almost all that salty stuff in cellophane bags is starchy, right? Potato chips, corn chips, pretzels, cheese curls—all are very bad news.

There is an exception: pork rinds. Americans have come to think of pork rinds as the worst possible junk food, but really they're about the most nutritious thing in the snack aisle. One ounce of potato chips has 152 calories with 10 grams of fat, 15 grams of starchy carb, 1 gram of fiber, and 2 grams of protein. One ounce of tortilla chips has 152 calories with 7 grams of fat, 18 grams of starchy carb, 2 grams of fiber, and 2 grams of protein. Pork rinds have a similar calorie and fat count—an ounce has 155 calories and 9 grams of fat. But they have *no* starch at all, and 17 grams of protein! That's more than two eggs. This could explain why I always could eat a whole bag of potato chips but fill up after I eat just four or five pork rinds.

Pork rinds come in a few flavors, including barbecue and salt and vinegar. But you can flavor your own. You can also run plain pork rinds through your blender or food processor for starch-free "crumbs," good for breading things.

Chee-Fauxs

For all you cheese puff lovers!

5 ounces pork rinds
¼ cup cheddar cheese powder, or to taste

Simply open the bag of pork rinds, add the cheese powder, roll down the top of the bag, and shake till the rinds are evenly coated.

Nutrient information: 5 servings, each with 155 calories, 9 g fat, 17 g protein, 0 g carbohydrate, 0 g dietary fiber

Note: This analysis is for the rinds only; total carbohydrate and calorie count will depend on what brand of cheddar cheese powder you buy. Barry Farm brand, available in 1-pound bags through Amazon.com, has 8 grams of carbohydrate per ¼ cup. This would bring the carbohydrate count per serving to 1.6 grams.

Sweet Cinnamon Crunchies

You're going to think I'm nuts, but these are surprisingly good. If you're jonesing for a sweet and crunchy snack—caramel corn or the like—try these.

¼ cup Splenda
¼ teaspoon cinnamon
5 ounces pork rinds

In a small dish, stir together the Splenda and cinnamon. Dump the mixture into your bag of pork rinds, roll down the top, and shake till they're evenly coated.

Nutrient information: 5 servings, each with 160 calories, 9 g fat, 17 g protein, 1 g carbohydrate, trace dietary fiber

Sauces and Gravies

Many sauces and soups, and all gravies, call for some sort of starchy thickener, usually flour, cornstarch, or arrowroot. These may be a minor source of starch in your diet, but if you eat a lot of stuff like this, it can add up. What to do?

There are a couple of great substitutes: *guar* and *xanthan*. As awful as they may sound, the truth is, you've been eating them all your life. Guar and xanthan are finely powdered fibers that are widely used as thickeners by the food-processing industry. They have no flavor—just like the starchy thickeners you've been using! You can buy guar or xanthan (they're interchangeable) at your local health food store.

Do *not* simply replace your starchy thickener with an equal amount of guar or xanthan! They are much more powerful thickeners. The easiest way to use these thickeners is to put one in an old salt shaker and keep it by the stove. When you want to thicken gravy, sauce, soup, or whatever, sprinkle your thickener lightly over the dish while whisking all the while. Stop when your dish is a little less thick than you want it to be; guar and xanthan continue to thicken on standing.

Unlike starchy thickeners, guar and xanthan do not need to be cooked to thicken, so you don't need to sauté the thickener in your drippings to make gravy. And you can use them to give a nice, rich thickness to smoothies and protein shakes.

17

The Art of Baking with Starch-Free Flours

by Dana Carpender

Baking is one of the most complex forms of cooking. It's not like making chili or soup, where a quarter cup more or less of chopped onion, or an extra few ounces of ground beef, won't make a big difference. Baking has to be reasonably precise to work.

Converting standard baking recipes into low-starch recipes is more complicated than converting other sorts of recipes and requires a variety of different ingredients. It's not as simple as saying, "Instead of a cup of flour, use a cup of X." There is no one ingredient I've found that works well as a one-for-one substitution for flour or for other starchy ingredients, like cornmeal.

But there's a bonus: added flavor. Starch, as Dr. Rob has told you, is flavorless. If you doubt it, put a pinch of plain white flour on your tongue. See? Nothing. The ingredients we're going to use instead all actually taste good! Trust me, this does *not* hurt the flavor of the finished product!

So let's talk a little about what flour does and what ingredients can replace it. First, some baseline stats: 1 cup of all-purpose flour contains 95 grams of carbohydrate (starch), 3 grams of fiber, and 13 grams of protein. In baked goods, flour serves two main functions: volume and structure.

Volume

Quite a lot of what flour does in baked goods is very simply to make up volume. Indeed, many recipes have been developed simply to turn flour, a flavorless paste, into something palatable. It's best to make up the volume of baked goods with a combination of ingredients. Here are the ones I use most often:

• **Almond meal.** You can buy almond meal preground in the baking aisle of most big grocery stores. I make my own: I buy shelled almonds in bulk and run them through my food processor using the S-blade. All the recipes in this book that call for almond meal will work with either store-bought or homemade almond meal. Store your almond meal in a snap-top container.

• **Pumpkin seed meal.** I started baking with pumpkin seed meal after readers with nut allergies asked what they could substitute for almond meal. I have yet to have a recipe using pumpkin seed meal not work out, and I've yet to hear of a pumpkin seed allergy. Furthermore, pumpkin seeds are cheaper than almonds and more nutritious. You can buy shelled pumpkin seeds in bulk at health food stores. You can also find them at Latin American markets, where they will be labeled pepitas.

Make pumpkin seed meal the same way you make almond meal. Store it in a snap-top container. Almond meal and pumpkin seed meal are generally interchangeable in my recipes.

• **Flaxseed meal.** Don't bother making flaxseed meal. The little suckers are just too tough for the average food processor to handle. It's easier just to buy flaxseed meal preground. Where I live, I can find flaxseed meal both at health food stores and in the baking aisle of big grocery stores. I use Bob's Red Mill Golden Flaxseed Meal.

While whole flaxseeds keep a long time, they go rancid quite quickly after they're ground. Buy your flaxseed meal from a store with a high turnover, and store it in the freezer.

Flaxseed meal is high in soluble fiber, so it holds moisture in baked goods. It has a mild, pleasant, nutty flavor.

• **Wheat bran.** You get a lot of fiber from wheat bran: 1 cup of wheat bran contains 37 grams of carbohydrate, of which 25 grams are fiber! Wheat bran can be used for adding bulk and volume to baked goods without a lot of starch. It also adds a wheaty taste.

• **Wheat germ.** Wheat germ has more starch than bran but far less than flour: 1 cup of wheat germ contains 60 grams of carbohydrate, with 15 grams of fiber. It also is a good source of protein (27 grams in that cup), valuable oils, and several B vitamins. Again, it adds a wheaty flavor to baked goods. I buy raw wheat germ at my health food store, or you can use the toasted wheat germ in the cereal aisle at the grocery store.

• **Oat bran.** The amount of starch in oat bran is close to the amount in wheat germ: 1 cup of oat bran contains 62 grams of carbohydrate, with 14 grams of fiber. It adds a nice flavor to many baked goods and helps hold moisture. Oat bran is also good as a binder in meat loaves in place of bread crumbs or crushed cereal—I usually use about one-fourth to one-third of the amount of crumbs or cereal called for in the original recipe.

• **Vanilla whey protein powder.** Available at GNC, health food stores, or wherever bodybuilding supplements are sold, vanilla whey protein powder has a mild vanilla flavor that works well in many baked goods. It also supplies one of the best, most easily assimilated forms of protein available, making your baked goods nutritious and satisfying. Because vanilla whey protein is more powdery than nut or seed meals and has a slightly sticky quality when wet, it helps your baked goods hold together. I often start

204 Low-Starch Cuisine: Discovering a Tastier Way to Eat

with a combination of equal parts of vanilla whey and almond meal when substituting for flour in cookies or quick breads; this is a good combination for many things.

The brand I like is Designer Whey French Vanilla, which I get at GNC, but I have used several different brands of vanilla whey protein powder. So long as it has no added sugar—read the ingredient list—it should be fine.

- **Rice protein powder.** Made by a company called Nutribiotic and available through health food stores, rice protein is useful for savory recipes where vanilla won't fit. If your health food store doesn't carry this, they can order it for you. Substitute unflavored whey protein, if you prefer.

Structure

Although mainly starch, wheat flour (both whole wheat flour and white flour) contains small amounts of protein, mostly in a form called *gluten*. Gluten is what makes bread and other yeast doughs stretchy, so that they can blow up like a billion tiny balloons as the yeast multiplies and creates carbon dioxide. This is how yeast bread rises. Gluten also keeps cookies, crackers, and quick breads from being too delicate and crumbly.

It is difficult to make good yeast bread while eliminating gluten and starch both; I'm afraid I have no substitute if you are gluten intolerant.

What I have used in a few of these recipes is pure, separated wheat gluten, sometimes called "vital wheat gluten." I buy Bob's Red Mill brand, which I get in the baking aisle at my big grocery store or at my health food store. What wheat gluten lacks in starch, it makes up for in protein: 1 cup has just 12 grams of carbohydrate and 1 gram of fiber but 189 grams of protein!

Sweeteners

While these are primarily low-starch recipes, I've also kept the sugar content low. I confess to a long-standing, gut-level distrust of sugar. I've used Splenda sweetener for a lot of the sweetness, with just enough carbohydrate-containing sweetener to get the textures right.

These recipes use Splenda Granulated (or the store brand versions), which is measured the same as sugar. Splenda in packets is far sweeter and cannot be substituted one-for-one.

I simply cannot bring myself to use white sugar. I have, instead, generally called for Sucanat—unrefined sugarcane juice that has simply been dried and ground up into a coarse powder. Sucanat tastes like brown sugar, but it contains all the vitamins and minerals that are removed from sugar. It's still sugar, but at least it's not completely nutritionally vacant. Sucanat is available at health food stores.

If you like, you can substitute granulated sugar or brown sugar for Sucanat. If you'd like to lessen the blood sugar impact of these recipes still further, you can substitute a polyol (sugar alcohol) sweetener like maltitol, xylitol, erythritol, or DiabetiSweet for Sucanat or sugar where it's called for. (If you use xylitol, be aware that it is profoundly toxic to dogs. Don't let your four-footed friends steal a cookie!)

The recipe analyses always are for the first sweetener listed.

The Cost of Specialty Ingredients

Yes, everything listed here is more expensive than flour, some of it much more so. Of course, it is also far more nutritious than flour. And unfortunately, since flour is what's making you sick, it will never be cheap for you again. In short, cheap starchy food is a luxury you can no longer afford.

And remember, since these ingredients are all high in protein, fat, fiber, or some combination of the three, they are *filling*. You will find yourself satisfied with two pancakes or a single slice of toast. And instead of feeling hungry again a couple of hours later, you're going to be full for a long, long time. That means less money spent on junk from vending machines and convenience stores, which you shouldn't be eating anyway.

Let's get to some recipes!

Buttermilk Pancake and Waffle Mix

If you're a pancake or waffle fan, make this up and keep it on hand. Then on Saturday or Sunday morning, when you've got time, make a double or triple batch of pancakes or waffles, and stash the extras in the refrigerator to warm up on busy weekday mornings.

> 1 cup dried buttermilk powder
> 2 cups vanilla whey protein powder
> 1½ cups pumpkin seed meal
> ¼ cup flaxseed meal
> ¼ cup wheat germ
> 4 teaspoons baking powder
> 2 teaspoons baking soda
> 1 teaspoon salt
> ¼ cup Splenda Granulated

Simply measure all ingredients into a big mixing bowl, and use your whisk to stir it up till everything is very evenly blended. Store in a snap-top container in your fridge or freezer. (You could use a big zipper-lock bag, but it's far easier to scoop the mix out of a snap-top container.)

Nutrient information: 16 servings (about 4½ cups total), each with 192 calories, 5 g fat, 27 g protein, 12 g carbohydrate

Pancakes from Buttermilk Pancake and Waffle Mix

With crisp bacon, these are the perfect Sunday breakfast!

1½ cups Buttermilk Pancake and Waffle Mix
1 egg
½ cup water

First put a big skillet or griddle over medium heat. The temperature of your cooking surface is important; when I used too cool a pan, the pancakes took a long time to brown and were dry. A good guide is one drop of water dripped on the cooking surface: it should skitter around, rather than sitting there (too cool) or simply evaporating (too hot.)

Measure your pancake mix into a mixing bowl, and add the egg and water. Stir with a whisk just until you're sure no pockets of dry stuff remain.

Scoop the batter with a ¼ cup measure, and cook as for regular pancakes (flip them when the edges look dry). Serve hot with butter and your choice of sugar-free pancake syrup, Splenda and cinnamon, or low-sugar preserves.

Nutrient information: 4 servings (2 pancakes per serving), each serving with 288 calories, 8 g fat, 39 g protein, 17 g carbohydrate, 4 g dietary fiber

Waffles from Buttermilk Pancake and Waffle Mix

You'll see that this recipe doesn't make a lot—just four waffles in my waffle iron. But using this recipe for the proportions, it's easy to double, triple, or even quadruple your batch.

1 cup Buttermilk Pancake and Waffle Mix
½ cup water
1 egg
¼ cup melted butter

Preheat your waffle iron. Don't even start mixing stuff till you have it plugged in.

Measure your Buttermilk Pancake and Waffle Mix into a mixing bowl.

In a separate bowl, whisk together the water, egg, and melted butter. When your waffle iron is hot and ready to cook, dump the egg and butter mixture into the dry stuff, and whisk it up, just till no pockets of dry stuff are left.

Bake immediately, according to the directions that come with your waffle iron. Serve with butter and your choice of sugar-free pancake syrup, cinnamon and Splenda, low-sugar jam or jelly, or another topping of your choice.

Nutrient information: Approximately 4 waffles, each with 299 calories, 17 g fat, 26 g protein, 12 g carbohydrate, 3 g dietary fiber

Note: For super light and crispy waffles, separate the egg, and whip the white stiff. Set the egg white aside while you add the wet ingredients to the dry. Then, once you've stirred up your batter, fold in the whipped egg white just before baking. This method makes great waffles, but I seldom want to do that much work before breakfast!

Zucchini Bread

Moist and sweet yet substantial, a slice of this bread with a cup of tea is sheer heaven and will keep you full and energetic for hours.

  1 pound zucchini
  ¼ cup Sucanat or sugar or polyol sweetener, divided
  ½ cup coarsely chopped walnuts
  1 cup almond meal
  ¾ cup vanilla whey protein powder
  ¼ cup flaxseed meal
  ½ cup Splenda
  1 teaspoon baking soda
  1 teaspoon baking powder
  ½ teaspoon salt
  ¼ cup plain yogurt
  2 large eggs
  1 tablespoon lemon juice
  6 tablespoons melted butter

Preheat your oven to 375°F, placing a rack in the middle position. Spray a 9 inch × 5 inch loaf pan well with nonstick cooking spray, and then use a tiny bit of flour or a little extra almond meal to "flour" the pan, tapping out any excess. (Alternatively, you could use one of the nonstick sprays that include a little flour, like Baker's Joy.)

Using the shredding disk of your food processor or your box grater, shred your zucchini, and put it in a big nonreactive bowl. Sprinkle it with 1 tablespoon of the Sucanat or sugar, and toss, then sprinkle it with another tablespoon of Sucanat or sugar, and toss again. Let this sit while you continue assembling your bread.

Spread your chopped walnuts on a baking sheet. Slide them into the oven, and set your timer for 5 to 7 minutes. (Don't skip the timer, or you'll burn 'em, sure as you're born.)

While the nuts are toasting, assemble the almond meal, vanilla whey protein powder, flax meal, Splenda, baking soda, baking powder, salt, and the rest of the Sucanat or other sweetener in a mixing bowl. Use a whisk to stir the dry ingredients together till everything's well distributed.

The timer went off! Pull the nuts out, and throw 'em in with the dry ingredients. Give the whole thing another stir.

In a separate bowl or a big glass measuring cup, whisk together the yogurt, eggs, lemon juice, and melted butter. Set aside for a moment.

Remember that zucchini you shredded? A fair amount of liquid will have drained off of it by now. Drain it well, squeezing it a bit with clean hands to get extra moisture out.

Now dump the zucchini and the yogurt-egg mixture into the dry ingredients, and use a whisk to quickly combine everything, stirring just until there are no pockets of dry stuff left. Scrape the batter into your prepared loaf pan, and smooth the top with your rubber scraper if you think it needs it. Put it on a center rack in the oven, and set a timer for 30 minutes.

When the timer goes off, turn the pan around (this helps it bake evenly), and give it another 30 minutes. Test with a wooden toothpick or skewer in the center. It should come out clean.

Cool your zucchini bread in the pan for 10 to 15 minutes, and then turn it out on a wire rack to finish cooling.

Wrap it in a plastic bag or plastic wrap. Store it in the refrigerator.

Nutrient information: 15 slices, each with 204 calories, 14 g fat, 13 g protein, 10 g carbohydrate, 3 g dietary fiber

Coconut Loaf

After all the brouhaha about saturated fats, it turns out that coconut and its ultrasaturated oil are really, really good for you; they improve thyroid function, stimulate the immune system, and even appear to lessen the risk of heart disease. So eat coconut and coconut products without fear or guilt. This loaf would be good as a tea bread for breakfast but is sweet enough to be a dessert, too. A little whipped cream wouldn't hurt, either!

> 1 cup almond meal
> 1 cup vanilla whey protein powder
> ½ cup Splenda
> 2 tablespoons Sucanat or sugar or polyol sweetener
> 1 teaspoon baking powder
> ¼ teaspoon ground cinnamon
> 1 pinch ground cloves
> ½ teaspoon salt
> 1⅓ cups shredded coconut meat
> 2 teaspoons butter
> 2 teaspoons coconut oil
> ½ cup coconut milk
> ¼ cup milk or half-and-half
> 2 eggs

Preheat the oven to 350°F. Butter a 3½ inch × 7 inch loaf pan, or coat the pan with nonstick cooking spray. Cut a piece of foil, waxed paper, or baking parchment to fit the bottom, and line the bottom of the pan. Butter or spray the foil or paper, too. Put a tablespoon or two of almond meal in the pan, and shake the pan to coat the paper or foil, and up the sides a bit. Set aside.

In a mixing bowl, combine all the dry ingredients—almond meal, vanilla whey protein powder, Splenda, Sucanat, baking powder, cinnamon, cloves, salt, and coconut. Stir together until all ingredients are evenly distributed.

Melt the butter and coconut oil together. Add the coconut milk and milk. Now add the eggs, and stir it all together. Pour the liquid mixture into the dry ingredients, and stir until all ingredients are moistened.

Pour the batter into your prepared pan. Bake for 40 to 45 minutes, or until a toothpick inserted in the center comes out clean. Cool in the pan for 5 to 10 minutes, and then run a knife around the edge to loosen the bread. Tip it out on a wire rack to finish cooling.

Nutrient information: 10 slices, each with 250 calories, 13 g fat, 24 g protein, 11 g carbohydrate, 2 g dietary fiber

Note: Look for unsweetened shredded coconut at your local health food store. It keeps well if you put it in a snap-top container, so feel free to buy enough to last for a couple of months. Your health food store may well have coconut oil and coconut milk, too. If not, try the international aisle of a big grocery store, with the Indian or Thai foods. You might also check Asian markets. If you can't find either one, you can substitute butter and milk.

Banana Nut Bread

Not only does this version of an old, familiar favorite have the starch removed, it also has as much protein per slice as two eggs. That means a slice of this bread with a cup of coffee makes a breakfast that staves off hunger till lunch.

1 tablespoon flour
1¼ cups chopped walnuts
1 cup almond meal
⅞ cup vanilla whey protein powder (1 cup minus 2 tablespoons)
2 tablespoons vital wheat gluten (If you're gluten intolerant, you can leave this out and increase the vanilla whey protein to 1 cup.)
½ cup Splenda
¼ cup Sucanat
¾ teaspoon baking soda
¼ teaspoon salt
3 bananas, very ripe and soft (Mine were dark brown all over!)
¼ cup plain yogurt
2 large eggs
6 tablespoons butter, melted

Preheat oven to 350°F. Spray a 9 inch × 5 inch loaf pan with non-stick cooking spray, and dust it with the flour. (Alternatively, you can use a nonstick spray with flour included, like Baker's Joy.)

Spread the walnuts in a shallow pan, and slide them into the oven. Set the timer for 5 to 7 minutes.

While your walnuts are toasting, measure the almond meal, vanilla whey protein, wheat gluten, Splenda, Sucanat, baking soda, and salt into a mixing bowl. Stir everything together till the ingredients are all evenly distributed. (When the timer goes off, get your nuts out of the oven!)

In a second bowl, mash the bananas well. Add the yogurt, eggs, and melted butter, and whisk all of this together. Dump the banana mixture into the dry ingredients and fold it in, using a rubber scraper, cutting all the way down to the bottom of the bowl. After the first couple of strokes, add the walnuts, and continue mixing just until there are no big pockets of dry stuff left. Do not overmix! Scrape the batter into your prepared loaf pan.

Bake for 50 to 60 minutes, or until a toothpick inserted in the center comes out clean and the loaf is pulling away from the sides of the pan a bit. Let the loaf cool in the pan for 5 to 10 minutes. Then carefully turn it out onto a wire rack to complete cooling. As soon as your bread is cool, wrap it in plastic wrap or a plastic bag.

Serve warm or at room temperature, either plain, with butter, or with—yum!—cream cheese.

Nutrient information: 15 slices, each with 258 calories, 16 g fat, 17 g protein, 14 g carbohydrate, 2 g dietary fiber

Cheese 'n' Green Onion Corn Bread

What a great side dish with ribs or chicken! If you like, you can leave out the cheese and onions for a plain, Southern-style corn bread to eat with butter and low-sugar preserves. And don't worry about that vanilla whey protein; for some reason, it doesn't clash with the onion-cheese flavor. I couldn't taste it at all.

⅓ cup whole-grain cornmeal
⅓ cup almond meal, homemade
⅓ cup flaxseed meal
1 cup vanilla whey protein powder
2 tablespoons Splenda or sugar
½ teaspoon salt
1 tablespoon baking powder
⅛ teaspoon cayenne (optional)
1 cup milk
⅓ cup melted coconut oil or peanut oil
1 large egg
½ cup sliced green onions
¾ cup shredded cheddar cheese, divided
1 tablespoon butter

Preheat oven to 400°F. While it's heating, put a 10-inch cast-iron skillet in the oven to heat, too.

In a mixing bowl, combing the cornmeal, almond meal, flaxseed meal, vanilla whey, Splenda or sugar, salt, baking powder, and cayenne. Stir these dry ingredients together until everything is evenly distributed.

Measure the milk, crack the egg into it, and whisk them together. Whisk the oil into the milk and egg mixture.

Now dump the liquid ingredients into the dry ingredients, and whisk it just until there are no pockets of dry stuff left. Now whisk in the green onions and ½ cup of the cheese.

Put on a really good oven mitt! Pull your very hot skillet out of the oven, and set it on the stove top (with no burners lit!) Give it a quick squirt of nonstick cooking spray. Now throw in the butter and slosh it around to cover the bottom of the skillet as it melts.

While the skillet is still smoking hot, pour in your batter. Put the skillet back in the oven, and set your timer for 25 minutes.

When the timer goes off, sprinkle the last ¼ cup of cheese evenly over the top of the corn bread. Return it to the oven, and let it bake for another 5 minutes.

Your corn bread should be done now! But stick a wooden toothpick or skewer in the center, and see if it comes out clean. If it does, it's done. If not, give it a few more minutes.

Serve hot, with plenty of butter.

Nutrient information: 8 wedges, each with 364 calories, 23 g fat, 30 g protein, 13 g carbohydrate, 5 g dietary fiber

Two-Bran Molasses Bread

This bread is utterly wonderful toasted and spread with butter. Don't have a bread machine? You can make this by hand, if you like. But I see bread machines at the Goodwill and at yard sales all the time—mine cost me $10 at a yard sale. Not a big investment!

⅓ cup oat bran
¼ cup wheat bran
3 tablespoons wheat germ
1 cup boiling water
1½ teaspoons molasses
1½ tablespoons Sucanat
½ cup almond meal
1 cup wheat gluten
⅓ cup vanilla whey protein powder
1 teaspoon salt
1½ tablespoons butter
1 envelope active dry yeast

Put the oat and wheat brans and the wheat germ in the bread case of your bread machine. Pour the boiling water over them, and let them sit until they're just warm—at least 20 minutes.

Add everything else in the order given, unless your machine gives far different instructions—if so, follow your machine's instructions as to the order.

Run your machine for a 1½-pound loaf on the whole wheat cycle. Remove the bread from the case promptly when done, and let it cool on a wire rack.

Nutrient information: 14 slices, each with 146 calories, 5 g fat, 19 g protein, 7 g carbohydrate, 2 g dietary fiber, 10 mg cholesterol

Note: The texture of your dough is vital. Let your bread machine run for 4 or 5 minutes, and then peek. The dough should be in

one cohesive ball. If it is too liquid and not forming a ball, add a tablespoon at a time of one of the dry ingredients, letting the machine knead it in before you add more. You want to add just enough so that the dough forms a ball. If your dough is too stiff, leaving dry stuff at the bottom of the bread case or breaking into lumps, add a tablespoon of water at a time, again, till you have a single cohesive dough ball.

When your dough has the correct texture, you can close the machine and let it do its thing.

Pizza Crust

For quick and easy pizza, try low-carb tortillas for crusts—they're quite good. But this recipe makes a real yeast-raised crust, for really truly pizza. I use Ragú Pizza Sauce (not Ragú Pizza Quick Sauce, which has corn syrup in it) and think it's quite good. If you live in the Chicago area, Pastorelli Italian Chef pizza sauce is the best I've tried.

> 1¼ cups water
> 1 cup wheat gluten
> 1 cup rice protein
> ½ cup oat bran
> ½ cup flaxseed meal
> ¾ cup almond meal
> 2 tablespoons extra-virgin olive oil
> 1½ teaspoons salt
> 1 envelope active dry yeast

Put all the ingredients in your bread machine in the order given, and run through the dough cycle. When it's done, punch it down, and let it rise one more time.

Divide the dough into two balls, and let it rest for 10 minutes. Using a rolling pin and your hands, roll, pat, and stretch your dough out to cover two pizza pans. If you don't have pizza pans, jelly roll pans (baking sheet with a small edge) work well. The dough will be quite elastic.

Preheat your oven to 450°F. Brush your crusts with a little extra olive oil, and then spread with pizza sauce. Top with mozzarella and/or provolone, and whatever toppings you like—Italian sausage (brown and crumble it first), pepperoni, Canadian bacon, sautéed peppers/onions/mushrooms, anchovies, and heck, pineapple if you like!

If you like a crisp crust, place your pan on the floor of the oven (you'll have to do your pizza in shifts if you do). Otherwise, you can just put it on the oven rack. Bake 8 to 12 minutes or until the cheese is bubbly and starting to brown. Serve with Parmesan, red pepper flakes, and oregano to sprinkle on top, the way they do at your favorite pizzeria.

Want pizza on a moment's notice? Make your crusts ahead of time and bake them for 5 to 6 minutes. Cool, wrap, and freeze. Then on a busy night when you want pizza, pull one out, grab a jar of pizza sauce, and go to town!

Nutrient information: For each slice of an 8-slice pizza (crust only), 204 calories, 9 g fat, 27 g protein, 8 g carbohydrate, 4 g dietary fiber

Brownies!

Moist, dense, fudgy, and oh-so-chocolaty!

¼ cup vanilla whey protein powder
¼ cup flaxseed meal
¼ cup almond meal
1 cup Splenda
½ cup sugar or polyol sweetener
½ cup unsweetened cocoa powder
1 pinch salt
¾ cup melted butter (1½ sticks)
3 eggs
1 teaspoon vanilla extract
¾ cup chopped walnuts or pecans (optional)

Preheat oven to 350°F. Spray a 9-inch square baking pan with nonstick cooking spray.

Measure the vanilla whey protein powder, flaxseed meal, almond meal, Splenda, sugar, cocoa powder, and salt into a bowl, and stir them with your whisk till everything is evenly distributed. (If you like, you can stop here and store this combination in a snap-top container in the fridge or freezer, as brownie mix. You can double, triple, even quadruple the recipe if you like, and when you want to make brownies, just measure out 2¾ cups of the mix.)

In a mixing bowl, whisk the melted butter, eggs, and vanilla together. Then whisk in the dry ingredients. Stir in the nuts, if using.

Spread the batter evenly in the prepared pan.

Bake for 20 to 25 minutes, or until it's just starting to pull away from the edges of the pan. Cool completely in the pan before cutting.

Nutrient information: 6 brownies, each with 201 calories, 15 g fat, 7 g protein, 12 g carbohydrate, 2 g dietary fiber

Butterscotch Oatmeal Balls

Oh, man. These are the best cookies I've come up with in quite a while.

> 1½ cups almond meal
> 2 cups vanilla whey protein powder
> 1 teaspoon baking soda
> ½ teaspoon cinnamon
> ½ teaspoon salt
> ¾ cup butter, softened
> 1 cup Splenda
> ½ cup Sucanat
> 2 eggs
> 1 teaspoon vanilla extract
> 1 cup rolled oats

Preheat oven to 350°F. Coat cookie sheets with nonstick cooking spray.

In a mixing bowl, measure and combine the almond meal, vanilla whey protein powder, baking soda, cinnamon, and salt. Stir together till everything is evenly distributed.

In another bowl, using an electric mixer, beat the butter, Splenda, and Sucanat together till the butter's fluffy and everything is very well combined. Beat in the eggs and vanilla, again combining very well.

Now add the dry-ingredient mixture, adding about one-third of the mixture at a time. When all of the dry ingredients are mixed in, add the oatmeal, and mix till it's evenly distributed.

Using clean hands, roll the dough into 1-inch balls, and place them on prepared cookie sheets. They don't spread a lot, so you can place them fairly close.

Bake for 8 minutes, and then cool on wire racks. This leaves the cookies soft and chewy on the inside. If you want crisp cookies, you can place them farther apart, flatten each one with a fork, and bake for a couple more minutes, but they're awfully good like this.

For a nice variation, chop ¾ cup of chocolate chips—regular or sugar-free—to a medium-fine consistency in the food processor, and stir them in with the oatmeal.

Nutrient information: 40 outrageously delicious cookies, each with 123 calories, 7 g fat, 10 g protein, 7 g carbohydrate, 1 g dietary fiber

Nadine's Miracle Bran Muffins

This recipe was in my book The Glycemic-Load Diet Cookbook. *I've also included it here because unless you're eating bran cereal regularly, it's hard to get adequate insoluble fiber in your diet. Most bran muffins don't have enough fiber in them to do you much good. Dr. Rob, his nurse Nadine, and some other good cooks have been working on this bran muffin recipe for six years to get it right. What's special about these muffins—aside from the fact that they're delicious—is that each one contains as much fiber as a bowl of All-Bran cereal. Don't omit the mashed yams. They're key to a moist texture.*

> 1½ cups All-Bran cereal
> 1 cup of almond meal or whole wheat flour
> 3 cups wheat bran
> 2 tablespoons brown sugar
> 1 teaspoon baking powder
> 1 teaspoon baking soda
> 2 teaspoons ground allspice
> 1 teaspoon cinnamon
> ½ teaspoon nutmeg
> ½ teaspoon salt
> ¾ cup dried cranberries
> 1 cup mashed canned yams or sweet potatoes
> ¾ cup chopped walnuts or almonds
> 4 eggs
> 1¼ cups milk
> ¼ cup water
> 1 cup unrefined safflower oil
> 1 teaspoon vanilla extract
> Butter for greasing the muffin cups

Adjust the oven rack to the lower-middle position. Preheat the oven to 350°F.

In a food processor with the S-blade in place, process the All-Bran until it has the texture of bread crumbs. Transfer to a large bowl. If you are using almond meal, process the almonds until they have the texture of cornmeal.

Add the almond meal (or flour) to the bowl along with the wheat bran, sugar, baking powder, baking soda, allspice, cinnamon, nutmeg, and salt. Stir to combine. Add the dried cranberries, yams, and nuts.

Break the eggs into another large bowl, and beat lightly with a fork. Add the milk, water, oil, and vanilla. Whisk to combine thoroughly.

Add about a third of the dry mixture to the egg-milk mixture, and mix thoroughly. Repeat until all the ingredients are used.

Coat the muffin cups generously with butter. Spoon the batter into the muffin cups, filling each to the rim. Bake until a toothpick inserted into the center of one of the muffins comes out clean or with a few moist particles adhering to it, about 20 minutes. Be careful not to overcook. Bran hardens if cooked too long.

Nutrient information: 12 muffins; with almond meal, each with 373 calories, 28 g fat, 13 g protein, 27 g carbohydrate, 9 g fiber; or with whole wheat flour, each with 360 calories, 26 g fat, 10 g protein, 31 g carbohydrate, 11 g fiber

18

A Seven-Day Low-Starch Meal Plan

Here's an illustration of what a low-starch eating style is like. This is essentially how I have been eating for the past ten years. You can see that it's not exactly deprivation. It includes some typical indiscretions (pizza on Tuesday, pasta on Friday) and ways you can mitigate the effects those slips have on your blood sugar.

Notice that by avoiding bread, potatoes, rice, and sugar-containing soft drinks and otherwise eating heartily, you can easily keep your daily glycemic load below 500.

MONDAY	GLYCEMIC LOAD
Breakfast	
1 whole orange	32
2 eggs	0
2 slices bacon	0
½ Nadine's Miracle Bran Muffin (Ch. 17)	50
Coffee	0

Snack
8-ounce latte	27
Apple	78

Lunch
Cobb salad (lettuce, turkey, avocado, bacon, blue cheese, vinaigrette dressing, no croutons)	15
Milk	27

Snack
Mixed nuts	15
Grapes	40

Dinner
Green salad (lettuce, tomato, avocado, blue cheese dressing)	20
½ barbecued chicken	0
Broccoli	15
Mashed Faux-tatoes (Ch. 16)	60
Butter	0
1 glass of red wine	0

Dessert
Dark chocolate, two 1-inch squares	25

Total Glycemic Load **411**

TUESDAY	GLYCEMIC LOAD

Breakfast
Yogurt, apple, fruit, bran, granola medley (see note below)	90
Coffee	0

Snack

8-ounce latte	27
Almonds	10

Lunch

Turkey, ham, and avocado tortilla wrap	80
Milk	27

Snack

Pear	57

Dinner

Green salad (lettuce, tomato, avocado, blue cheese dressing)	20
3 slices pizza with Italian sausage (cut away ⅔ of crust)	70
1 beer	0

Total Glycemic Load	**406**

Note: Add 3 heaping tablespoons unsweetened, full-fat yogurt to ½ bowl of chopped apple plus another fruit. Add ¼ cup bran and 1 tablespoon granola, and mix.

WEDNESDAY	GLYCEMIC LOAD

Breakfast

Walnut and bran cereal with strawberries (see note below)	90
Microwave omelet, 2 eggs	0
Coffee	0

Snack

8-ounce latte	27
2 plums	72

Lunch

Teriyaki stir-fried chicken and vegetables (no rice)	20
Tea	0
Fortune cookie	25

Snack

Cheese	0
Apple	78

Dinner

Caesar salad	20
Salmon	0
Asparagus	15
Cauli-Rice (see recipe in Ch. 16)	60
1 tablespoon butter	0
1 glass white wine	0

Dessert

Chocolate-covered almonds	30

Total Glycemic Load	**437**

Note: The only common, true deficiency in the American diet is that of insoluble fiber. By far the best source is All-Bran cereal. If you don't find bran cereal particularly exciting to eat, before you give up on it, buy a bag of chopped walnuts and add a heaping handful to your cereal. It changes the whole game.

THURSDAY	GLYCEMIC LOAD

Breakfast

Cottage cheese and chopped peach	67
Sliced ham	0
½ Nadine's Miracle Bran Muffin (Ch. 17)	50
Coffee	0

Snack
8-ounce latte	27
Mixed nuts	20

Lunch
Spinach salad with bacon and Parmesan crumbles and vinaigrette dressing	15
Baked cod	0
Coffee	0

Snack
Pear	57
Cheese	0

Dinner
Jalapeño peppers, olives, carrot, and celery appetizer	20
½-pound cheeseburger with lettuce, tomato, mustard, and mayonnaise on low-carb tortilla (see note below)	0
Grapes (1 cup)	40
Milk	0

Dessert
6 hot-cinnamon jelly beans	46

Total Glycemic Load	**481**

Note: Hamburger buns are loaded with starch. However, a wheat tortilla has a glycemic load of only 80, perfectly acceptable. Just wrap the tortilla around the hamburger patty and add the usual ingredients. It's a little sloppier than a hamburger bun, but it does the job.

FRIDAY	GLYCEMIC LOAD

Breakfast

Omelet with ham, cheese, mushrooms, onions	0
Pineapple slice	50
½ Nadine's Miracle Bran Muffin (Ch. 17)	50
Coffee	0

Snack

| 8-ounce latte | 27 |
| Apple | 78 |

Lunch

| Green salad | 0 |
| Hamburger with top bun removed | 100 |

Snack

| Mixed nuts | 15 |

Dinner

Green salad with tomato, avocado, vinaigrette dressing, and diced walnuts	0
1 cup spaghetti with meat sauce, with starch blocker acarbose, 100 mg (see note below)	113
Spinach steamed with butter and lemon juice	0
1 glass red wine	0

Dessert

| Strawberries | 13 |
| Dark chocolate, two 1-inch squares | 25 |

| **Total Glycemic Load** | **471** |

Note: The acarbose should lower the glycemic load by approximately one-third. Notice also the walnuts and vinegar in the salad, both of which are proven to reduce glycemic load. You can measure your blood sugar 2 hours afterward to see if the starch-blocking strategies worked.

SATURDAY	GLYCEMIC LOAD
Breakfast	
½ grapefruit	32
Egg frittata with mushrooms and sausage (see note below)	0
Coffee	0
Snack	
Orange	71
Lunch	
Chili, Texas style (no beans)	75
Milk	27
Snack	
Apple	78
Cheese	0
Dinner	
Caesar salad	20
Steak, 12 oz.	0
Broccoli	15
½ sweet potato	80
Butter	0
1 glass red wine	0
Dessert	
Raspberries and yogurt sweetened with ½ tsp. sugar	44
Total Glycemic Load	**442**

Note: Whip up any number of eggs in a bowl, and add whatever you want—sausage, mushrooms, bell pepper, etc. Pour into a greased skillet on medium heat until the bottom is firm, and then bake at 350°F until the top is firm.

SUNDAY	GLYCEMIC LOAD
Breakfast	
Maggie's Crustless Mini-Quiche (see recipe in Ch. 16)	0
½ Nadine's Miracle Bran Muffin (Ch. 17)	50
Coffee	0
Snack	
Apple	78
Cheese	0
Lunch	
Roast beef wrap (wheat tortilla)	80
Milk	27
Snack	
Mixed nuts	15
Grapes	40
Dinner	
Green salad (lettuce, tomato, avocado, blue cheese dressing)	20
Pork chops	0
Navy beans	0
Asparagus	40
Butter	0
Milk	27
Dessert	
Dark chocolate, two 1-inch squares	25
Total Glycemic Load	**411**

Appendix A

Metric Conversion Factors

Volume Measurement Conversions

U.S.	Metric
¼ teaspoon	1.25 ml
½ teaspoon	2.50 ml
¾ teaspoon	3.75 ml
1 teaspoon	5.00 ml
1 tablespoon	15.00 ml
¼ cup	62.50 ml
½ cup	125.00 ml
¾ cup	187.50 ml
1 cup	250.00 ml

Weight Conversion Measurements

U.S.	Metric
1 ounce	28.4 g
8 ounces	227.5 g
16 ounces (1 pound)	455.0 g

Cooking Temperature Conversions

Celsius/Centigrade: 0 degrees Centigrade and 100° Centigrade are arbitrarily placed at the melting and boiling points of water and are standard to the metric system.

Fahrenheit: Fahrenheit established 0° as the stabilized temperature when equal amounts of ice, water, and salt are mixed.

To convert temperatures in Fahrenheit to Celsius, use this formula:

$$C = (F - 32) \times 0.5555$$

So, for example, if you are baking at 350° Fahrenheit and want to know that temperature in Celsius, use this calculation:

$$C = (350 - 32) \times 0.5555 = 176.65 \text{ degrees Centigrade}$$

Appendix B

References

Aude, Y.W. et al. 2004. The national cholesterol education program diet vs. a diet lower in carbohydrates and higher in protein and monounsaturated fat: A randomized trial. *Archives of Internal Medicine* 164:2141–46.

Baer, D.J. et al. 1997. Dietary fiber decreases the metabolizable energy content and nutrient digestibility of mixed diets fed to humans. *Journal of Nutrition* 127(4):579–86.

Bond-Brill, J. et al. 2002. Dose-response effect of walking exercise on weight loss: How much is enough? *International Journal of Obesity Related Metabolic Disorders* 26(11):1484–93.

Brand-Miller, J.C. et al. 2003. Physiological validation of the concept of glycemic load in lean young adults. *Journal of Nutrition* 133(9):2728–32.

Bryner, R.W. et al. 1999. Effects of resistance versus aerobic training combined with an 800-calorie liquid diet on lean body mass and resting metabolic rate. *Journal of the American College of Nutrition* 18(2):115–21.

Cao, Y. et al. 2009. Effects of moderate versus lower fat diets on lipids and lipoproteins: A meta-analysis of clinical trials in subjects with and without diabetes. *Journal of Clinical Lipidology* 3:19–32.

Chiasson, J.L. et al. 2003. Acarbose treatment and the risk of cardiovascular disease and hypertension in patients with impaired glucose tolerance: The STOP-NIDDM Trial. *Journal of the American Medical Association* 290:486–94.

Di Meglio, D.P. and Mattes, R.D. 2000. Liquid versus solid carbohydrate: Effects on food intake and body weight. *International Journal of Obesity Related Metabolic Disorders* 24(6):794–800.

Ebbeling, C.B. et al. 2007. Effects of a low-glycemic load vs. low-fat diet in obese young adults: A randomized trial. *Journal of the American Medical Association* 297:2092–2102.

Flegal, K.M. et al. 2002. Prevalence and trends in obesity among US adults, 1999–2000. *Journal of the American Medical Association* 288:1728–32.

Fontaine, K.R. et al. 2003. Years of life lost due to obesity. *Journal of the American Medical Association* 289(2):187–93.

Foster, G.D. et al. 2003. A randomized trial of a low-carbohydrate diet for obesity. *New England Journal of Medicine* 348(21): 2082–90.

Foster-Powell, K., Holt, S.H.A., and Brand-Miller, J.D. 2002. International table of glycemic index and glycemic load values. *American Journal of Clinical Nutrition* 76:5–6.

Gerich, J.E. 2003. Contributions of insulin-resistance and insulin-secretory defects to the pathogenesis of type 2 diabetes mellitus. *Mayo Clinic Proceedings* 78:447–56.

Halton, T.L. et al. 2008. Low-carbohydrate-diet score and risk of type 2 diabetes in women. *American Journal of Clinical Nutrition* 87:339–46.

Hays, J.H. et al. 2003. Effects of a high saturated fat and no-starch diet on serum lipid subfractions in patients with documented atherosclerotic cardiovascular disease. *Mayo Clinic Proceedings* 78:1331–36.

Hodge, A.M. et al. 2004. Glycemic index and dietary fiber and the risk of type 2 diabetes. *Diabetes Care* 27:2701–2706.

Howard, B.V. et al. 2006. Low-fat dietary pattern and weight change over 7 years: The Women's Health Initiative Dietary Modification Trial. *Journal of the American Medical Association* 295:39–49.

Irwin, M.L. et al. 2003. Effect of exercise on total and intra-abdominal body fat in postmenopausal women: A randomized controlled trial. *Journal of the American Medical Association* 289(3):323–30.

Jarvi, A.E. et al. 1999. Improved glycemic control and lipid profile and normalized fibrinolytic activity on a low-glycemic index diet in type 2 diabetic patients. *Diabetes Care* 22(1):10–18.

Joline, W.J. et al. 2007. High dietary glycemic load and glycemic index increase risk of cardiovascular disease among middle-aged women: A population-based follow-up study. *Journal of the American College of Cardiology* 50:14–22.

Lavin, J.H. et al. 2002. An investigation of the role of oro-sensory stimulation in sugar satiety. *International Journal of Obesity Related Metabolic Disorders* 26(3):384–88.

Liu, S. et al. 2000. A prospective study of dietary glycemic load, carbohydrate intake, and risk of coronary heart disease in US women. *American Journal of Clinical Nutrition* 71:1455–61.

Manson, J.E. et al. 2002. Walking compared with vigorous exercise for the prevention of cardiovascular events in women. *New England Journal of Medicine* 347(10):716–25.

Mattes, R.D. and Rothacker, D. 2001. Beverage viscosity is inversely related to postprandial hunger in humans. *Physiological Behavior* 74(4–5):551–57.

Miyatake N. et al. 2002. Daily walking reduces visceral adipose tissue areas and improves insulin resistance in Japanese obese subjects. *Diabetes Research in Clinical Practice* 58(2):101–107.

National Center for Health Statistics. 2001. Third National Health and Nutrition Examination Survey. http://www.cdc.gov.

Nielsen, V.N. and Joensson, E. 2006. Low-carbohydrate diet in type 2 diabetes: Stable improvement of bodyweight and glycemic control during 22 months of follow-up. *Nutrition and Metabolism* 3:22.

O'Keefe, J.H. and Cordain, L. 2004. Cardiovascular disease resulting from a diet and lifestyle at odds with our paleolithic genome: How to become a 21st-century hunter-gatherer. *Mayo Clinic Proceedings* 79:101–108.

Packianathan, I.C. et al. 2002. The eating disorder inventory in a UK National Health Service obesity clinic and its response to modest weight loss. *Eating Behavior* 3(3):275–84.

Pasman, W.J. et al. 2003. Effect of two breakfasts, different in carbohydrate composition, on hunger and satiety and mood in healthy men. *International Journal of Obesity Related Metabolic Disorders* 27(6):663–68.

Pelkman, C.L. et al. 2004. Effects of moderate-fat (from monounsaturated fat) and low-fat weight-loss diets on the serum lipid profile in overweight and obese men and women. *American Journal of Clinical Nutrition* 79:204–212.

Pereira, M.A. 2002. Dairy consumption, obesity, and the insulin resistance syndrome in young adults: The CARDIA study. *Journal of the American Medical Association* 287(16):2081–89.

Pereira, M.A. et al. 2004. Effects of a low-glycemic load diet on resting energy expenditure and heart disease risk factors during weight loss. *Journal of the American Medical Association* 292(20):2482–90.

Petersen, K.F. et al. 2004. Impaired mitochondrial activity in the insulin-resistant offspring of patients with type 2 diabetes. *New England Journal of Medicine* 350:664–71.

Pittas, A.G. et al. 2005. A low-glycemic load diet facilitates greater weight loss in overweight adults with high insulin secretion but not in overweight adults with low insulin secretion in the CALERIE Trial. *Diabetes Care* 28:2939–41.

Ryden, A. et al. 2003. Severe obesity and personality: A comparative controlled study of personality traits. *International Journal of Obesity Related Metabolic Disorders* 27(12):1534–40.

Samaha, F.F. et al. 2003. A low-carbohydrate as compared with a low-fat diet for severe obesity. *New England Journal of Medicine* 348(21):2082–90.

Schulze, M.B. 2004. Sugar-sweetened beverages, weight gain, and incidence of type 2 diabetes in young and middle-aged women. *Journal of the American Medical Association* 292(8):927–35.

Shai, I. et al. 2008. Weight loss with a low-carbohydrate, Mediterranean or low-fat diet. *New England Journal of Medicine* 359:229–41.

Slentz, C.A. et al. 2004. Effects of the amount of exercise on body weight, body composition, and measures of central obesity. *Archives of Internal Medicine* 164:31–39.

Sparti, A. et al. 2000. Effects of a diet high or low in unavailable and slowly digested carbohydrates on the pattern of 24-hour substrate oxidation and feelings of hunger in humans. *American Journal of Clinical Nutrition* 72(6):1461–68.

Sturm, R. 2003. Increases in clinically severe obesity in the United States, 1986–2000. *Archives of Internal Medicine* 163:2146–48.

Taylor, R. 2004. Causation of type 2 diabetes: The Gordian knot unravels. *New England Journal of Medicine* 350:639–41.

Tuomilehto, J. et al. 2004. Coffee consumption and risk of type 2 diabetes mellitus among middle-aged Finnish men and women. *Journal of the American Medical Association.* 291(10):1213–19.

United States Department of Agriculture, Agricultural Research Service. 2004. National Nutrient Database for Standard Reference, Release 17. Nutrient Data Laboratory home page, http://www.nal.usda.gov/fnic/foodcomp.

Van Wymelbeke, V. et al. 2004. Influence of repeated consumption of beverages containing sucrose or intense sweeteners on food intake. *European Journal of Clinical Nutrition* 58(1):154–61.

Warren, J.M. et al. 2003. Low glycemic index breakfasts and reduced food intake in preadolescent children. *Pediatrics* 112(5):e414.

Watkins, L.L. et al. 2003. Effects of exercise and weight loss on cardiac risk factors associated with Syndrome X. *Archives of Internal Medicine* 163:1889–95.

Westerman, E. et al. 2008. The effects of a low-carbohydrate, ketogenic diet versus a low-glycemic diet on glycemic control in type 2 diabetes mellitus. *Nutrition and Metabolism,* DOI: 10.1186/1743-7075-5-36.

Westerterp, K.R. and Kester, A.D. 2003. Physical activity in confined conditions as an indicator of free-living physical activity. *Obesity Research* 11(7):865–68.

Appendix C

Websites and Suggested Reading

The website supplement to *The Low-Starch Diabetes Solution* is lowglycemicload.com. You will find additional information on foods as well as useful articles to help you manage your diabetes, cholesterol, and weight. You can also submit questions and comments about losing weight or managing your type 2 diabetes.

Suggested Reading

The Glycemic-Load Diet by Rob Thompson, M.D. (McGraw-Hill, 2006). More about the low-glycemic load approach to weight loss.

The Glycemic-Load Diet Cookbook by Rob Thompson, M.D., and Dana Carpender (McGraw-Hill, 2009). 150 low-glycemic-load recipes with tips on low-glycemic-load shopping and eating.

Good Calories, Bad Calories by Gary Taubes (Alfred A. Knopf, 2007). An excellent analysis of the evolution of current scientific thinking about diet.

"International table of glycemic index and glycemic load values: 2002," by Kaye Foster-Powell, Susanna H. A. Holt, and Janette C. Brand-Miller (*American Journal of Clinical Nutrition*, volume 76 [2002], pages 5–56). This is the largest compilation of glycemic loads available. To compare the glycemic loads in the table with the ones in this book, multiply the ones in the table by 10. You may have to adjust the serving sizes in the tables, because some of them are different from typical American serving sizes. You can download a copy from the journal's website, www.ajcn.org.

Other Websites

www.americanheart.org/profilers
An interactive tool provided by the American Heart Association for helping people make informed decisions about preventing and treating high blood cholesterol, high blood pressure, and several heart conditions.

www.holdthetoast.com
An excellent source for low-starch meals and snacks by Dana Carpender, author of *The Glycemic-Load Diet Cookbook* and *500 Low-Carb Recipes from Snacks to Desserts the Whole Family Will Love*.

Index